Writing your Nursing Portfolio

Writing your Nursing Portfolio
A Step-by-Step Guide

Fiona Timmins and Anita Duffy

 Open University Press

Open University Press
McGraw-Hill Education
McGraw-Hill House
Shoppenhangers Road
Maidenhead
Berkshire
England
SL6 2QL

email: enquiries@openup.co.uk
world wide web: www.openup.co.uk

and Two Penn Plaza, New York, NY 10121-2289, USA

Published in association with Nursing Standard and RCN Publishing.

First published 2011

A catalogue record of this book is available from the British Library

ISBN-13: 978-0-33-524284-9
ISBN-10: 0-33-524284-7
eISBN: 978-0-33-524285-6

Library of Congress Cataloging-in-Publication Data
CIP data applied for

Typeset by RefineCatch Limited, Bungay, Suffolk
Printed in the UK by Bell & Bain Ltd, Glasgow

Fictitious names of companies, products, people, characters and/or data that may be
used herein (in case studies or in examples) are not intended to represent any real
individual, company, product or event.

Mixed Sources

Product group from well-managed
forests and other controlled sources
www.fsc.org Cert no. TT-COC-002769
© 1996 Forest Stewardship Council

FSC

The *McGraw-Hill* Companies

Contents

PRAISE FOR THIS BOOK

"I am delighted to endorse this practical and accessible guide to writing and developing a portfolio for nurses. Unlike many 'how-to-do' approaches to portfolio compilation, this book acknowledges the complexity involved in learning from practice, and recording that learning in a meaningful way. The book respectfully guides the reader through essential elements to be considered if a portfolio is to be more than a depository of paper, yet avoids prescription in acknowledging the individual nature of the portfolio and its necessity to reflect the nurse's own journey through their career."

Professor Melanie Jasper, Head of College of Human and
Health Sciences, Swansea University, UK

"This book is intended for nurses at all stages of their careers and offers a much-needed step-by-step guide to planning, writing and maintaining a portfolio. I was particularly pleased to see a strong emphasis on reflection and education, as a means of encouraging nurses to think critically and learn from their own practice. All in all, this is a very well-constructed book which I highly recommend."

Professor Gary Rolfe, Swansea University, UK

Dedication

To all the great teachers that we have come across in our lives, the best of whom are our children, Kerry-Anne and Nathan Timmins, Jack and Robbie Duffy.

'Go raibh maith agaibh as éisteacht linn, ár bpáistí áille. Ba mhaith linn éisteacht níos mó libhse.'

Acknowledgement

We would like to acknowledge Ms. Caroline Ivory for her contributions to the development of reflective pieces included.

Developing your portfolio

1

By the end of this chapter you will:

○ Understand the term 'portfolio' and other associated terms such as 'mind-mapping', 'reflective friend', 'reflexivity', 'learning style', 'continuous professional development' (CPD) and 'e-portfolio'.
○ Be aware of portfolio development in nursing and the history of nursing portfolios.
○ Understand why you need to develop a portfolio.
○ Understand where you need to start.

In this introductory chapter we will begin to explore what is meant by a portfolio, and what you might expect a portfolio to contain. The chapter explains the basic requirements for portfolio development, and begins to demonstrate how you can develop and structure your own nursing portfolio.

Whether you are working as a healthcare assistant, a student nurse, a newly-qualified nurse or have many years of clinical experience, at some stage of your nursing career you may choose or be required to engage in portfolio development and reflect on your nursing practice. Many nurses feel unsure about beginning a portfolio. However, most say that once they begin the process and engage with a facilitator or group to reflect on their practice, they find it enjoyable and beneficial. The majority of nurses are proud of the learning they have achieved once they have completed their portfolio.

Who is this book for?

This book is written for all nurses wanting to engage in portfolio development regardless of whether or not they are currently undertaking further education. This chapter presents an overview of the crucial elements of getting started on a portfolio and provides a step-by-step approach to help you begin and continue to develop your portfolio. As time goes by you will be able to expand on your portfolio and use it for promotional opportunities, performance appraisal, and personal and professional development. Moreover, during the process of reading this book you should develop self-awareness and self-assessment skills, as you become increasingly aware of your strengths and weaknesses.

The portfolio

The term 'portfolio' comes from the Latin *portare*, meaning 'to carry' and *foglio*, meaning a 'sheet'. So in its most basic interpretation, a 'portfolio' is a *receptacle for information*. In nursing a portfolio is more than just a record of continuous professional development (CPD) containing certificates, diplomas and other relevant documents; rather, it is a collection of *evidence* summarizing what you have learned from prior experience through reflection.

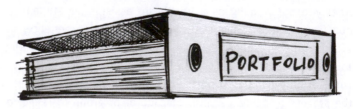

In other words, portfolios are more than simple collections of documents that demonstrate learning achievements. A nursing portfolio provides evidence of previous experience and presents a dynamic record of your growth and professional learning over time. A portfolio is also an *account of learning* based on practice and critical reflection: 'A portfolio is a ... cohesive account of work-based learning that contains relevant evidence from practice and critical reflection on this evidence. Its primary purpose is to 'display achievement of professional competence or learning outcomes and knowledge development' (Timmins 2008: 115).

It is this more comprehensive interpretation that will be used throughout this book. We will also use the term 'professional portfolio' to denote that its function relates to your *professional role* as a nurse. While you may be quite comfortable with the notion of recording your attendance at study events, courses and programmes in your portfolio along with any certificates or awards you have received, you may feel that the prospect of *reflecting on your achievements* is a daunting one. In fact, the demonstration of learning achievements through reflection is often a cause for concern and uncertainty for practising nurses; and yet the skills of reflection and critical thinking are deemed crucial by the Nursing and Midwifery Council (NMC 2004). It is believed that thinking about and reflecting on your practice, and developing a portfolio as a result, makes your learning more explicit as you translate your clinical experiences into documented evidence. You can then learn to critically examine the nature of your learning in relation to specific experiences in your nursing practice and demonstrate that you have learned from those experiences and how you have achieved or maintained your clinical competence as a result. Although undergraduate nursing students are required to develop portfolios in the UK (NMC 2004), your experience in this field may have been insufficient to prepare you to do so.

Portfolios are also very useful for 'unpacking' 'invisible' learning in the clinical arena, as well as helping you to maintain elements of ongoing clinical competence and accountability in relation to your nursing practice. They have been viewed as a vehicle for demonstrating reflective skills, critical thinking skills, decision-making skills, problem-solving skills and interpersonal communication skills, as well as indicating your array of clinical skills (Twadell and Johnson 2007).

Throughout this book we aim to improve your confidence with portfolio use. We will emphasize the importance of you, as a nurse, developing a portfolio. We will you take you through a step-by-step process so that you will be able to showcase your development as a professional nurse in a cohesive and concrete way as you travel from novice to expert in nursing practice.

Pause for Thought

- Consider the drawbacks of using a portfolio just to collect information about your professional experience and accolades. What are the advantages of using a portfolio in this way (just to contain information)?

- Consider the drawbacks of developing a more in-depth portfolio, one that critically reflects upon your professional experience and accolades, and includes more detailed information about you as a professional. What are the advantages of using a portfolio in this way (in-depth portfolio with critical reflection)?

Origins

During the last decade the term 'portfolio' has become very familiar in nursing education and practice. Portfolios were first used in nursing schools in the early 1980s (Cole *et al.* 1995) as a means of demonstrating – and more importantly evaluating – learning through establishing evidence of holistic learning achievements. Professional bodies in nursing practice have embraced the portfolio 'movement' and recommend that nurses maintain and develop a portfolio as part of their professional development. As mentioned earlier, in the UK nurses are expected to maintain a profile as a means of demonstrating CPD and this can form part of your professional profile. CPD is linked to the registration updating process in the UK through the Post-Registration Education and Practice (PREP) standards. The portfolio development process thereby symbolizes an important part of work-based learning (NMC 2008). The concept of 'work-based' or 'practice-based' learning is one that is well documented in the educational and nursing literature (see e.g. Quinn 1998; Gopee 2005) and can be demonstrated through the development of a professional portfolio.

Getting started

Pause for Thought

- Consider what you think you might need to include in your portfolio. Write everything down in a list.

- What aspects of your nursing practice do you think will inform the development of your portfolio?

- What other aspects of nursing practice might you need to think about before embarking on portfolio development?

Considering there is no correct way to organize and develop your portfolio you may find yourself overwhelmed before you have even begun. Some authors argue that portfolios do not conform to templates and any attempt to standardize your portfolio would not do you or your portfolio any justice and may even curtail your creativity (Hughes and Moore 2007). However, we hold the view that, especially for the novice portfolio developer, it is critically important that you have a framework to help you structure your portfolio in a logical and coherent manner. We will include more discussion about this as the book progresses. However, for the moment, a little brainstorming is needed. Take a moment to consider everything that you think your portfolio *should* contain.

You may have provided a vast range of responses to the earlier exercise, and it is important to consider your own personal views of the portfolio – after all it is a very individualized document, with no set format. The important elements that we think need to be considered are outlined in the 'mind-map' shown in Figure 1.1.

In order to successfully begin to develop your portfolio you will need to spend some time considering what nursing means to you, and some pointers are shown in Figure 1.1. You may wish to consider your *philosophy of nursing*, or that of the department or organization within which you work. You may think about including some of your CV (your whole CV is unlikely to be appropriate for a nursing portfolio as it will include non-relevant items such as sporting interests and other activities, such as your proficiency at the piano and so on: the portfolio must focus clearly on your learning achievements as a *nurse*).

Reflection (discussed in detail in Chapter 2) is paramount to the portfolio development process. Specifically, *critical reflection* is a conscious and deliberate strategy aimed at understanding and learning from clinical practice. Critically learning from and evaluating your nursing experience is one of the implicit aims of critical reflection. The lessons you learn from reflection can then be applied to your practice, providing a tangible link between theory and practice. In Chapter 2 we discuss the process of reflection and explain why it is such an important element of your portfolio. We describe a simple model of reflection that will guide you through your reflection on practice; and following this we hope that you will be in a good position to choose a model of reflection that suits you best for use in your portfolio.

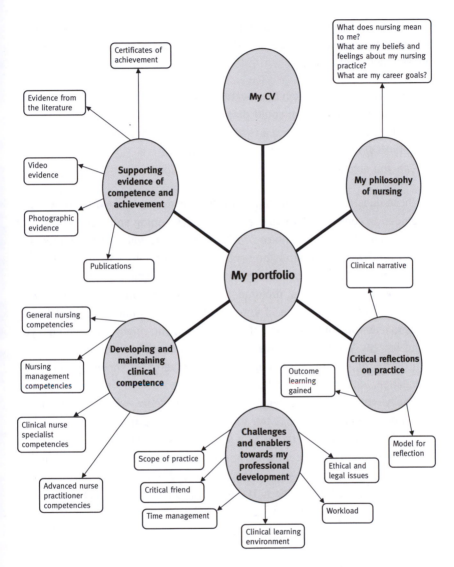

Figure 1.1 A mind-map of the important elements to consider when embarking upon portfolio development.

During your initial brainstorming session you may also consider what challenges and enablers there are in terms of your portfolio of professional development. For example:

- Does your workload seem to prevent you from getting started on a portfolio?
- Are there ways that you could plan your time better?
- Could you approach your manager to get some protected time within your duty to work specifically on your portfolio?
- Can you engage a reflective friend to assist you?

All these questions (and others) are worth considering and writing down. You also need to consider how you are currently developing and maintaining your clinical competence. Your choice of methods for this will ultimately affect the way in which your portfolio is presented. If, for example, you are attending a programme of study, your learning within this programme and your achievements (grades, certificates, diplomas) may be an important element in your portfolio. On the other hand, if you are attending a random range of locally or nationally run courses, relevant to your area, you might examine how you could link the learning you have gained from attending these to your reflection on the development of your ongoing competence, knowledge and skill acquisition, within your portfolio.

Finally, consideration of what constitutes *evidence* within a portfolio is extremely important. It is not the intention of the portfolio to merely house everything that you own; rather, you should be selective in the evidence you collect or retain. Evidence must be relevant and must fit with your portfolio's themes. For the most part evidence should be *objective*. For example, an attendance certificate for a training day on managing aggression and violence in the workplace is objective evidence that you attended. Your simply reporting that you attended (without the certificate) is not. On the other hand, evidence generated from your reflections will, by its very nature, be *subjective*. However, you can support your reflections with objective evidence (such as certificates of achievement and so on) to further strengthen your conclusions.

All of this initial brainstorming may take a little time, and it is worth noting your thoughts down in a notebook or journal. This phase is designed to get you thinking about important elements that may form part of your portfolio.

Brainstorming over, you need to consider whether your portfolio is for professional and personal development purposes or for academic purposes. If your portfolio is part of a programme of study it may have different requirements to the professional portfolio of the type we describe in this book. In an academic setting you will usually receive detailed instructions for your portfolio. However, there will still be many common elements between your academic portfolio and a professional one, so it is still worth reading on!

A step-by-step approach

It is important that when embarking on a major task, such as developing a portfolio, you break the task down into *manageable steps*. This section describes taking a step-by-step approach to your professional portfolio and a summary of these steps is outlined in the list below.

1 *Decide to engage in the process:* the first and most vital step!
2 *Commit:* a good way to do this is to declare your intention to a chosen 'reflective friend' (see below).
3 *Explore:* use this book to consider different types of portfolio and methods of reflection.
4 *Identify:* pinpoint the approach that works best for you, along with potential barriers to success. Consider how you will overcome such barriers.
5 *Negotiate:* group discussions and reflection are very useful. Discuss your thoughts and decisions so far with colleagues or a reflective friend. Always be open to ideas and suggestions others make for improvement.
6 *Plan:* now plan your strategy based on *realistic targets*.
7 *Implement:* begin to implement your strategy in a disciplined manner.
8 *Re-examine:* as you progress, periodically question and examine your personal attitudes and values.
9 *Persist:* no matter what barriers fall in your way, stay determined, persist, and you will succeed.

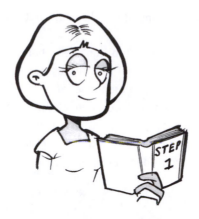

Decide to engage in the process

You may be required to develop a nursing portfolio as part of a nursing programme or perhaps you need to develop one for registration purposes or for personal and professional development reasons. Whatever the reason, when starting a portfolio it is important to plan how you will approach the process in a methodical manner.

A portfolio has a beginning and a middle, but may have no end. As you engage in the process you will find yourself on a journey of self-development and discovery and furthermore, as you continue to evaluate and learn from your practice, your personal and professional development and your portfolio will develop as a result. The 'end', therefore, will be the *product*. However, even after you've reached the 'end', your journey will continue, especially if your aim is to develop both personally and professionally.

In order to get started you might consider using a framework or a 'mind-map' (All and Havens 1997; Baugh and Mellott 1998), as shown in Figure 1.1. This should help you to structure your portfolio, decide what information you need to gather and include, and consider how you intend to present the portfolio. Mind-maps are a useful tool to develop critical thinking, challenge your thinking process and enable you to bridge the theory–practice gap. Furthermore, they are useful in helping you think critically about your clinical practice and synthesize your ideas, thereby facilitating meaningful learning.

Commit

Declaring your intention to develop a portfolio to a friend early on in the process not only helps you to visualize your goal, it also demonstrates self-determination. Having a 'reflective friend' (Bond and Holland 1998; Duffy 2008) is extremely useful because we are often so close to our own actions that we cannot see things clearly. For example, what is familiar and obvious to you may appear quite unique and unusual to a friend, and perhaps worthy of special attention in your portfolio. A reflective friend can assist you by supporting your reflections and interpretations of actions, attitudes, perceptions and beliefs in order to develop your portfolio entries.

A reflective friend can help you visualize alternative perspectives that you may not have realized on your own, and can change both you and your practice positively. However, you do need to choose this person carefully. You will be divulging very personal information and thus the wrong choice could lead to you ending up feeling self-critical, under-confident and defensive about your practice. What type of person makes a good reflective friend? A harmonious relationship is essential, therefore there needs to be a good 'match' between your personalities. You need to feel at ease with one another and have a mutual respect, both as nurses and as individuals. Carl Rogers (1961) considered the types of personal characteristic required of a facilitator. While the focus of the reflective friend is not necessary to facilitate your learning, these personal attributes, when present in the facilitator, bring out the best in the other person. For this reason they are useful to consider in the context of choosing your reflective friend. They are:

- Openness
- Curiosity
- Flexibility
- Supportiveness
- Consistency
- Self-disclosure
- Attentiveness
- Non-defensiveness
- Reliability

- Approachability
- Concern
- Trustworthiness
- Self-awareness
- Congruency
- Empathy

Pause for Thought

- Using Rogers' characteristics listed above, consider what personal characteristics you might wish to find in your reflective friend.

- What is the most critical personal characteristic that your reflective friend should have?

- Who would you consider being a suitable friend for you to choose?

- Why would you choose this person?

- Does this friend have all the personal characteristics in your list?

The scenario below examines this part of the process a little further. Josephine has decided to develop her professional portfolio, and needs to choose a reflective friend to assist her through the process.

Scenario: Josephine

Josephine is a 34-year-old staff nurse with six years' clinical experience in surgical nursing. The position of Junior Nurse Manager (F Grade) on the unit has been advertised and Josephine would like to apply for the position. She decides to develop her professional portfolio to demonstrate her clinical competence and ability to manage the unit in the absence of a more senior manager. She recalls a number of incidents that she could potentially reflect on to highlight her clinical competence in nursing management, writes about these and decides that she would benefit from the help of a reflective friend. She wants to develop her listening skills but is in a dilemma regarding the most suitable person to assist her in critiquing her practice. She narrows her choice down to two people:

- *Jane is a 45-year-old registered nurse working part-time on the unit. She has over 15 years' experience in nursing, has worked in two hospitals in the UK and has substantial life experience. Her husband died in a motorbike accident seven years before and her responsibilities include twin sons and a daughter, all attending secondary school. Jane has not advanced her nursing education since qualifying as a registered nurse because she feels she is too busy with life. Josephine often asks Jane's opinion on issues relating to her personal life and takes Jane's advice on most issues. She feels she can trust Jane.*
- *Maria is a new staff nurse on the unit; she started working on the surgical ward a month before. She had two years' nursing experience as a theatre nurse before she accepted the*

position of staff nurse in the surgical unit. Maria undertook a postgraduate diploma in theatre nursing and during the programme was required to develop a reflective portfolio. She is a quiet, very relaxed person. From Josephine's observations she appears to be a very professional practitioner. However, the two nurses work opposite shifts and Josephine does not know Maria very well at the moment.

Questions

- Who should Josephine choose as a reflective friend to help her develop her portfolio? Why?
- Who should Josephine not choose? Why?

Suggested answers

- Because Josephine is developing her portfolio for promotional purposes she needs to be strategic about choosing her critical friend. She could in fact ask *both* of these people to assist her. Jane would be an ideal critical friend if she has the time to commit to the process. She demonstrates the essential qualities necessary and has the clinical knowledge to assist Josephine. Her nursing experience is vast, not to mention her life experience, so she will be able to empathize with Josephine. Josephine trusts Jane's opinions and advice and is likely to respect her feedback. In addition, because guided reflection is a *two-way process* Jane may become more motivated to undertake further education and training herself.
- Maria may also have some of the qualities necessary to act as a reflective friend, but because the two nurses have not as yet built a trusting relationship she would not at this stage be the ideal candidate for Josephine. Nonetheless, as Maria has developed an educational portfolio Josephine could seek her advice about using a reflective cycle and writing up and presenting a portfolio.

Whoever they may be, your reflective friend should be someone who will motivate and encourage you to pursue your portfolio development within a supportive but challenging relationship.

Explore

After deciding on your reflective friend you are ready to move to the next step of the portfolio development process. There are essentially two formats available for you to develop your portfolio. The first is the *paper portfolio* and the second is the *e-portfolio*.

The paper portfolio

This is probably the simplest way: essentially, all you need is a ring binder and some dividers to structure your portfolio in an organized manner. Endacott *et al.* (2004) discuss various types of paper portfolio, and these are outlined in more detail in Chapter 4. Briefly though, they are:

- the shopping trolley model;
- the toast rack model;
- the spinal column model;
- the cake-mix model.

With the 'shopping trolley' model you simply place all your documents in any fashion into your portfolio. In the 'toast rack' model you organize the content of your portfolio in a more structured manner by using dividers. However, there is still no connection between the sections of the portfolio. The 'spinal column' model improves on this by introducing an over-arching theme – for instance, 'achieving competence in communication skills', which would be a likely theme for Josephine to choose for her portfolio. Finally, the most advanced model is the 'cake-mix', whereby the nurse builds the portfolio based on an over-arching narrative and links theory to practice through reflexivity. This is the model you would expect to see an advanced nurse practitioner use. However, this book will focus on developing your portfolio to at least the level of the 'spinal column' model. Your portfolio will then have a structure and an over-arching theme in relation to building and maintaining your clinical competence in your nursing practice.

E-portfolios

Alternatively, if you are competent at web-based work, you could choose to build an e-portfolio. An e-portfolio has been defined by eportfolio portal (2004) as a web-based information management system that uses electronic media and services. The e-portfolio 'movement' has developed as a result of three main factors: the dynamic nature of learning; the rapid growth of knowledge; and the changing needs of the healthcare environment. An e-portfolio is a digital version of a paper portfolio, whereby you collect and demonstrate your work and provide a record of evidence to show your achievement of clinical competence and professional growth over a period of time (Banks 2004). Nursing e-portfolios can include all the elements of a paper portfolio, such as your CV, evidence of clinical and research skills, evidence of management and leadership skills, evidence of further education, evidence of your use of a recognized reflective framework and case reports, lists of published work and details of research projects, with the useful addition of video and audio records.

E-portfolios are similar to personal websites and are context rich: you can upload digital evidence (e.g. photos, videos, scanned documents), thereby presenting a greater range of material data than in a paper portfolio. Further advantages of creating an e-portfolio are that the exercise will help to develop your information technology (IT) skills and you will be able to scan or search your documents quickly and easily. In addition, e-portfolios are very easy to access from any computer connected to the internet, anywhere in the world, providing more opportunities to share your work with mentors, colleagues and potential employers, both for performance appraisal and accreditation purposes. The power of technology allows rapid archiving and offers a range of useful tools to present your work in different formats. E-portfolios also encourage collaboration as you can easily share information and reflections with others. With the advances in technology in healthcare, the e-portfolio is likely to quickly become an established means of maintaining professional accountability and demonstrating professional and personal development in nursing practice.

However, it is not within the remit of this book to explain the process of setting up an e-portfolio, as our focus is on the paper portfolio. Clearly, all the techniques and strategies described in the following pages apply equally well to an e-portfolio, and if you are interested in developing such a portfolio further information can be found at www.pebblepad.co.uk/definitions.asp and http://mahara.org

Identify

You have now decided on your reflective friend and on the format you intend to use for your portfolio. You now need to spend some time identifying your *style* of learning. This will help you to work effectively with your reflective friend and to plan well for the task ahead. Learning styles can be categorized into four types, shown in Table 1.1.

Table 1.1 The four learning styles

Diverger	<ul><li>Prefers to observe rather than act</li><li>Good at coming up with ideas</li><li>Has a vivid imagination</li><li>Has a sensitive nature</li></ul>
Assimilator	<ul><li>Rational in nature</li><li>Good problem-solver</li><li>Technical</li><li>Displays difficulties with social interaction</li></ul>
Converger	<ul><li>Logical</li><li>Concise</li><li>Theoretical rather than practical</li><li>Solution-finder</li><li>Displays difficulties with social interaction</li></ul>
Accommodator	<ul><li>Practical</li><li>Intuitive</li><li>Enjoys challenges</li><li>Learns from practice</li><li>Weak analytical skills</li></ul>

You may find, after you have worked through the Learning Styles Inventory presented in Table 1.2, that you are more suited to one style than another, or perhaps your learning style is a combination of one or more styles. Whatever your strongest category may be, it is also important to identify your weakest category and work towards balancing your learning style in order to balance your learning. The Learning Styles Inventory is derived from an experiential theory and model of learning developed by Kolb (1984) and is based on the contributions of Dewey, Lewin and Piaget, three educational psychologists. It is a practical self-assessment instrument that will help you to assess your unique learning style, and only takes 30–45 minutes to complete. Try it out!

So how can this information help you to learn more effectively? Knowing your learning style will:

- Make you aware of your preferred style of learning, which you can then use to your advantage when learning new skills. For instance, do you learn better by doing or observing? Do you need structure to learn, or do you prefer to be creative?
- Motivate you to learn more effectively and achieve your learning goals.
- Expand on the *way* you learn by encouraging you to learn in new ways and not just using your preferred style. Try developing a relationship with someone whose learning style is different from your own and who can offer a different perspective on your learning and help you to develop a more balanced approach to the way you learn.
- Help you to work on your weaknesses and develop your learning and problem-solving skills in a holistic manner.
- Enable you to use your learning strengths to make better decisions and choose better courses of action to solve problems.
- Help you to change your learning habits or study skills to fit with your learning style.
- Make you more self-aware. By recognizing your strengths and weaknesses you will become more confident in your ability to learn and hence boost your learning potential.

Table 1.2 Learning Styles Inventory

Place in rank order each set of four words shown below. Assign a '4' to the word which best characterizes your learning style, a '3' to the next best, a '2' to the next and a '1' to the least characteristic word. Do not 'tie' any words: every word in each line must be assigned a different score from 1–4.

1	___ involved	___ tentative	___ discriminating	___ practical
2	___ receptive	___ impartial	___ analytical	___ relevant
3	___ feeling	___ watching	___ thinking	___ doing
4	___ accepting	___ aware	___ evaluating	___ risk-taker
5	___ intuitive	___ questioning	___ logical	___ productive
6	___ concrete	___ observing	___ abstract	___ active
7	___ present-oriented	___ reflecting	___ future-oriented	___ practical
8	___ open to new experiences	___ perceptive	___ intelligent	___ competent
9	___ experience	___ observation	___ conceptualization	___ experimentation
10	___ intense	___ reserved	___ rational	___ responsible
(for scoring only)	___ (CE)	___ (RO)	___ (AC)	___ (AE)

Now add all of your scores in each column. The sum of the first column gives you your score on 'concrete experience' (CE); the second column gives you your score for 'reflective observation' (RO); the third column gives you your score for 'abstract conceptualization' (AC); and the final column is your score for 'active experimentation' (AE). Now transfer your scores to the Learning Style Profile below (Figure 1.2) by placing a mark by the number you scored on each of the four dimensions. Connect these four marks with straight lines – the resulting diagram should look like a kite and gives you the profile of your learning style.

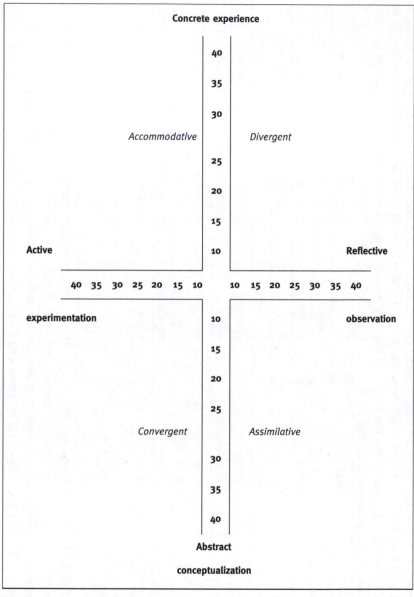

Figure 1.2 Learning Style Profile.

Negotiate

An extension of working with your reflective friend is to use *peer learning* or *learning in groups*. Some nurses find this very helpful in assisting with reflection on professional practice. Having numerous perspectives can aid understanding. Learning occurs through active engagement with peers and colleagues who may have experienced similar incidents and can empathize with and understand the issues that have caused you concern.

In *group reflective sessions* ground rules are imperative. These should include issues related to reflector confidentiality, mutual respect for members of the group, time limits per reflection and discussions to allow the expression of emotions. Furthermore, engaging a reflective model, which will be discussed in detail in Chapter 2, can enable critical analysis of incidents by the group.

It is important to understand that reflections with others may not always proceed smoothly (Duffy 2008); therefore, group facilitators must be prepared to manage any challenges as they arise. Group reflections are often difficult to begin with. However, many clinical practice areas undertake group reflection and evidence from the literature reveals positive results (see e.g. Bailey and Graham 2007).

In order to prepare for group reflection, the facilitator must recognize their own strengths and weaknesses and know when to gently encourage the reflector to express both positive and negative feelings, and, very importantly, recognize when the reflector is *not* ready to move on. In these situations, the facilitator should be confident enough to adjourn the group session, giving the individual the opportunity to return to reflecting on the incident at a later date, once he or she has had an opportunity to consider the issues in greater depth. Important ground rules that should generally be observed in group reflection include the following (Bailey and Graham 2007; Duffy 2008):

- *Protected time* should be allocated for guided reflective sessions.
- *Confidentiality* must be agreed by group members (unless, of course, unethical and unprofessional practice issues are reported).
- Group members should have *unconditional positive regard and respect* for each other.

- *The agenda should be prepared in advance* and sometimes it is useful to undertake ice-breaking exercises to encourage the group to feel at ease with each other.
- Each individual must take responsibility for their own learning, either as a guide or as a reflector.
- If there are more than two people reflecting in the session, each individual should be given an opportunity to speak and to receive feedback from their peers.

Plan, implement, re-examine and persist

The final steps of the process require time for practice and commitment to develop your reflective portfolio. Even though you are critically examining your nursing practice and clinical competence, portfolio development should be an enjoyable experience, both cathartic and empowering. Once you plan and begin the process and witness your journey of self-development you will probably find yourself more prepared to deal with future clinical incidents as a consequence of reflecting on your practice. You will become more self-aware and more confident of your clinical competence. If you return to your reflections as you progress through your portfolio, you will notice your professional and personal development over time. Portfolio development is like most skills in that the more you practise the better you become, and the more energy you give to your critical reflections on practice and development of your clinical competence the more your clinical competence and professionalism will develop. Once you see this change emerging, you should feel more encouraged to sustain the process.

Overcoming obstacles

Once you have decided to develop your nursing portfolio, and having read this introductory chapter, you are probably aware of the challenges that might present as obstacles on this journey of self-development. Write down some challenges that you think you might face and try to come up with some possible solutions.

Challenges	Solutions

In addition to the issue of choosing a reflective friend, dealt with in this chapter, above, some of the other challenges that might concern you at this stage will be addressed later on in this book. For example:

- choosing a reflective model that suits you (see Chapter 2);
- deciding how to structure your portfolio in a systematic manner (see Chapter 4);
- overcoming ethical or legal issues that may be inherent in a portfolio entry (see Chapter 5);
- choosing a critical incident that is worthy of inclusion in your portfolio (see Chapter 6);
- deciding which competency underpins a reflection entry (see Chapter 6).

You need to have some knowledge of the nursing competencies that you are expected to achieve in order to demonstrate clinical competence. You are also expected to know how to use a model of reflection (discussed in Chapter 2), and how to search the literature to assist you in linking theory to practice before you can begin to develop an evidence-based reflective portfolio.

Conclusion

You should now have some idea of the process involved in developing your reflective portfolio, be it for personal reasons, to critique your clinical practice, to demonstrate your achievement of clinical competence, to learn more about yourself as a practising clinician or to engage in portfolio development as a requirement of an academic programme.

Summary

- The development of a portfolio is a *process* not a discrete task.
- The portfolio process is a journey of both personal and professional development.
- Engaging a reflective friend can be of huge benefit.
- The process may seem daunting, but start with small steps and begin with the 'end' in mind.

References

Au, A.C. and Havens, R.L. (1997) Cognitive/concept mapping: a teaching strategy for nursing, *Journal of Advanced Nursing*, 25: 1210–19.

Bailey, M. and Graham, M. (2007) Introducing guided group reflective practice in an Irish palliative care unit, *International Journal of Palliative Care*, 13(10): 550–60.

Banks, B. (2004) *E-portfolios: their uses and benefits. A White Paper* (version 1.1), www.excellencegateway.org.uk/media/ferl_and_aclearn/ferl/resources/organisations/fd%20learning/e-portfoliopaper.pdf (accessed on 5 September 2010).

Baugh, N.G. and Mellott, K.G. (1998) Clinical concept mapping as preparation for student nurses' clinical experiences, *Journal of Nursing Education*, 37(6): 253–6.

Bond, M. and Holland, S. (1998) *Skills of Clinical Supervision for Nurses*. Maidenhead: Open University Press.

Cole, D., Ryan, C. and Kick, F. (1995) *Portfolios Across the Curriculum and Beyond*. Thousand Oaks, CA: Corwin Press.

Duffy, A. (2008) Guided reflection: a discussion of the essential components, *British Journal of Nursing*, 17(5): 334–9.

Endacott, R., Gray, M.A., Jasper, M., McMullan, M., Miller, C., Scholes, J. and Webb, C. (2004) Using portfolios in the assessment of learning and competence: the impact of four models, *Nurse Education in Practice*, 4(4): 250–7.

eportfolio portal (2004) www.danwilton.com/eportfolios (accessed on 8 June 2010).

Gopee, N. (2005) Facilitating the implementation of lifelong learning in nursing, *British Journal of Nursing*, 14(14): 761–7.

Hughes, J. and Moore, I. (2007) Reflective Portfolios for Professional Development, in *Teaching Portfolio Practice in Ireland, A Handbook*, HEA/TCD/AISHE. Dublin: Centre for Academic Practice and Student Learning (CAPSL), Trinity College.

Kolb, D.A. (1984) *Experiential Learning*. Englewood Cliffs, NJ: Prentice Hall.

NMC (Nursing and Midwifery Council) (2004) *Standards of Proficiency for Pre-registration Nursing Education*. London: NMC.

NMC (Nursing and Midwifery Council) (2008) *Standards to Support Learning and Assessment in Practice. NMC Standards for Mentors, Practice Teachers and Teachers*. London: NMC, www.nmcuk.org/Documents/Standards/nmcStandards ToSupportLearningAndAssessmentInPractice.pdf (accessed on 9 May 2010).

Quinn, F. (1988) *The Principles and Practice of Nurse Education*. Cheltenham: Stanley Thornes.

Rogers, C. (1961) *On Becoming a Person: A Therapist's View of Psychotherapy*. London: Constable.

Timmins, F. (2008) *Making Sense of Portfolios: An Introduction to Portfolio use for Nursing Students*. Maidenhead: Open University Press.

Twadell, J. and Johnson, J. (2007) A time for nursing portfolios: a tool for career development, *Advances in Neonatal Care*, 7(3): 146–50.

Reflection

2

In this chapter we will explore the process of developing a reflective portfolio. The chapter explains the concept of reflection and the role of critical reflection in portfolio development.

What is reflection?

Reflection and reflective practice may be familiar terms to you.

Pause for Thought

● Write down any words or phrases that you associate with reflection and reflective practice.

You may have noted phrases such as 'looking back on' or 'looking inwards' when you considered the term reflection. 'Reflective practice' means thinking about these concepts in relation to your nursing. You may have considered terms like 'professional development' and 'improving practice'. If so then you are already very familiar with what these terms mean in this context.

However, if you were a little hesitant with your personal definitions, or found that you were immediately turned off the chapter based on your previous experiences of reflection, don't worry: such feelings are common. For some nurses the idea of reflection is a little too vague and for others it can be difficult to see where reflection fits into nursing practice. During the course of this chapter we will clarify these issues and introduce you to the skills required to incorporate reflection in your portfolio.

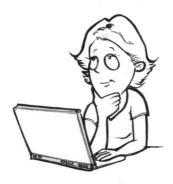

Reflection became a popular practice in nursing during the late 1980s and early 1990s. The writings of Donald Schön (1983) were very influential, as he described how professionals used reflection as a method of ongoing or continuous learning. Reflection could either be of an immediate reflexive nature, taking place during practice and referred to as *reflection in action*, or subsequent to it, known as *reflection on action*. Many nurses, mostly those in the academic community, embraced reflection as something that could be of benefit to nursing students and practitioners in terms of developing insight into professional practice through self-awareness. As a result, Schön's theories have been evident in much of the nursing literature over the last 30 or so years and a range of reflective models have been developed. Of particular interest here is the fact that reflection has become synonymous with portfolio development (McMullan *et al.* 2003).

In your work as a nurse you may have come across models of reflection as part of your coursework, as reflective frameworks are now commonly used in student assignments where consideration of practice is required. Or perhaps you have seen nursing students using models of reflection during clinical placements as part of their coursework, and they may have discussed this with you.

Reflection is a natural human thinking process of looking back over our actions, or situations that we have encountered that either caused us concern or gave us satisfaction. As nurses, due to the nature of our professional work, it is often necessary to reflect in order to plan for the future care of our patients, or due to a de-brief following a traumatic experience. In either case, the process of thinking back over events is not a new phenomenon to many practising nurses.

However, using a *model* of reflection to structure reflective thinking processes can be a new experience for many nurses and this process is not necessarily easy. You may be thinking, 'Well, if humans are naturally able to reflect on things, why do we need yet another model to complicate matters?' The answer is simple: models serve to formalize and make sense of your thinking processes. In particular, models help us to complete a *reflective cycle*: when we are left to our own reflective devices there may be a tendency to rehash a situation (either mentally or verbally to others) repeatedly without coming to any concrete solution or conclusion; by using a model of reflection you are enabled to systematically think through the event and are provided with opportunities to embrace new learning from the experience. Thus a *model of reflection* can be described as 'a complex and deliberate process of thinking about and interpreting experience in order to learn from it' (Boud *et al.* 1985: 135).

Partial journeys and Gibbs' model of reflection

The model of reflection developed by Gibbs (1988) is frequently used in nurse education settings, and you may be familiar with it already. The stages of this model are:

1   Describe the event
2   How does it make you feel (as a nurse)?
3   Evaluate: what was good or bad about the experience?
4   Analyse: what sense can you make of what happened?
5   Conclude
6   Action: what would you do differently in the future?

Although not moving beyond the descriptive phase in either this model or others is quite common in nursing, with practice, endurance and help from your reflective friend (see Chapter 1) you will find yourself beginning to evaluate and analyse your reflective journey as Gibbs' model suggests you should. Always bear in mind that using only selective parts of a model of reflection severely limits its usefulness in practice. This is especially true if you do not have a reflective friend to share your thoughts with. The tendency in this situation is to get caught in a cycle of thinking and feeling, with no solutions emerging. Without full use of your chosen reflective model, and without talking to your reflective friend, your thoughts and feelings may actually be misguided. You might for example reflect that you did a great job inviting relatives in to see their mother after her operation in a timely fashion, and cannot understand why they got angry with you. Full reflection, using a cycle and speaking with your reflective friend might inform you that you did not fully prepare the family for how pale their mother was or for all the tubes and wires they would see. Inappropriate reflections, such as this one, can result in:

● biased judgement towards yourself (either negative or positive);
● biased judgement towards others (either negative or positive);
● lack of personal progress to improve practice;
● a tendency towards conceit (believing you are right in situations where you may not have been);
● failure to understand the wider context;
● an inability to detach personal emotions from current reflection (e.g. if you have personal experience of the situation in your own life);
● failure to act;
● inappropriate personal emotional burden due to misplaced guilt.

This is not to say of course that simple outline descriptions of your practice, without reflection, don't have their place. There is value in using a diary to record personal experiences; similarly, *narratives* are used in practice, usually in research projects, to explore nurses' and patients' stories, and these too are valuable. However, we are concerned here with developing a structured portfolio and structured models of reflection are always a useful starting point. You may of course include personal stories and narratives in your portfolio as well, if you find these useful.

The breadth of reflection

An important thing to remember about reflection is that it doesn't have to relate to a specific incident. Reflection is often considered as being a one-off event, often referred to as a 'critical incident' in practice, whereby you think back over negative or positive experiences in order to understand what you could do differently or similarly the next time you encounter a comparable event. Real reflection, however, is much broader than this. In terms of your portfolio, using a model of reflection will enable you to tie the whole thing together. What you need is a flexible, yet comprehensive model of reflection, which you can use throughout your portfolio to unify its various elements. Thinking up specific practice episodes to reflect upon, while this has a place, is not the sole concern of the developing portfolio.

Why is reflection important?

Reflection is important in the context of portfolio development as it gives a structure to your thinking, right back across your career and all the learning that has unfolded. Using a model of reflection in your portfolio provides:

● An aide memoir documenting your achievements
● A structure upon which the whole portfolio is based

At the most basic level, reflection will help you to remember every element of your career that you wish to include in your portfolio, and will assist you in analysing your experience in more depth.

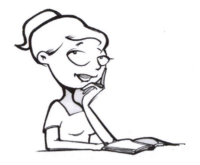

If you are a nurse who has been qualified for 12 months, at first you will probably find that your portfolio is rather sparse. It might look like this:

- Diploma in nursing 2006–2009, Walsbrook University
- Staff nurse, surgical ward, Bingley Hospital, 2009–present

Consequently, you may wonder exactly what needs to be put in next. At the back of your mind are the mandatory requirements of the need for 35 hours CPD evidenced within a profile before your next registration (NMC 2006). In addition, you may be considering a change of position to enhance your career, and therefore require a competitive portfolio or CV. In either case, your first attempt at thinking back over the last year can yield quite limited results. Two lines seem very little to describe the intense learning that you have experienced in the four years prior to now. This is where reflection comes into play.

Reflection on practice allows you to examine, explain, analyse and evaluate your specific learning from practice. In addition to outlining a more detailed portfolio of your experience, reflection will assist you in working out what your learning needs actually are. You will hopefully discover what it is you need to do next to achieve your personal goals or improve on your skills in practice. Furthermore, reflection can lead to your seeking out new learning opportunities, such as reading, taking a short course or attending relevant conferences.

Reflection on practice also helps you with your personal development planning – in other words, planning your career goals. You will begin to ask yourself some simple questions, such as:

- Where have I been?
- Where am I now?
- Where would I like to be?
- How will I get there?

Pause for Thought

- Write out your answers to these questions:

Where have I been?

Where am I now?

Where would I like to be?

How will I get there?

Reflection on competence requirements

Before we discuss the concept of reflection in a little more depth, it is worth taking a moment to consider the *core competencies* required for registration as a nurse in the UK (NMC 2010). These include:

- professional values;
- communication and interpersonal skills;
- nursing practice and decision-making;
- leadership, management and team working.

While these competencies are obviously quite broad, and more specific detail is available within the relevant documentation, they are very useful frameworks to guide both portfolio development, profiling and your own assessment of your learning needs.

Pause for Thought

- Consider one core competency that is relevant to your current practice that you might select to begin reflection on your learning.

- Why have you chosen that specific competency?

- Write down your strengths and weaknesses in relation to achieving this competency in your nursing practice.

If you are like many nurses, you may find that you have been collecting certificates, documents, articles and other items related to your ongoing professional development for years. You may have put these away in a cupboard or drawer for safe-keeping. For you, like others, the information is readily to hand should it be needed for PREP (NMC 2006) or other requirements. However, as time goes on you may become frustrated with your system, particularly as the number of artefacts gets greater. You may want to create a more organized system so that you can find items more quickly and, even more importantly, you may feel that the many documents undersell your valuable learning over the years and that there is more that you would like to add to explain matters, but you don't know how to go about this.

Using chosen competencies, such as the one you selected above, is a good way of organizing your achievements. Take a closer look at the competencies required and see whether or not your information could be categorized under some or all of these. Ultimately it is these set competencies that the NMC wish to see evidenced, and even though you may be engaged in a great deal more than this, you will find that the competencies are broad enough to permit many elements of practice to be included.

Once you have chosen a competence to begin with, you can begin the task of reflecting on your own achievements in relation to it. This reflection will help you to build a more in-depth portfolio as you select certain elements of your personal journey to examine and explain in more depth. To begin this process you need to know a little more about *how to reflect*.

How to start

Reflection should always begin at the *micro level*. For our nurse at the beginning of her career, her experience was as follows:

- Diploma in nursing 2006–2009, Walsbrook University
- Staff nurse, surgical ward, Bingley Hospital, 2009–present

In order to evaluate this cohesive, but brief, account consider presenting it in terms of themes, such as the domains of competence previously outlined. Begin by labelling these sub-themes within your portfolio, either as tabbed dividers in your binder, or as new files within your e-portfolio (portfolio structure will be covered in more detail in Chapters 3 and 4). Next you can begin to unpack and explore your work-based learning within these domains, both during your preparatory nurse education programme and since registration. These sub-themes are not of course set in stone. They may be less helpful for example if you have 25 years of nursing experience, in which case you might prefer to present your experiences under headings such as the areas in which you have worked. In either case, dividing your portfolio into sub-themes is extremely helpful for organizational purposes.

This is where the necessity for a model of reflection comes in. Without it your experiences simply turn into long lists or extremely extensive descriptions of what 'happened'. This approach (while it may have some relevance for you) is time consuming, and overall doesn't allow the function of the portfolio to prevail. You are trying to show evidence of your professional competence; that you are capable of critically reflecting upon the development or maintenance of that competence, and are able to provide a cohesive account of it. So you need to pick out *key events* from your experiences on which to reflect in depth.

To help you do this, there are numerous models of reflection available, and Rolfe *et al.* (2001) provide some good examples. But how do you choose which one is best for you?

Reflective models

The best reflective model is the one that most suits *you*, and it is by no means the case that 'one model fits all'. Duffy (2008) usefully presents what are known as the 'four Rs' of reflection, and these are a useful starting point: the Right guide, the Right model, Readiness and Reflexivity (i.e. 'reflecting on your reflections'). As we discussed in Chapter 1, a reflective friend is a hugely important (but not wholly essential) factor and that person (or indeed on a more formal level your clinical supervisor) will be able to assist you in choosing the right model. You also need to be ready for the consequences of the reflection that emerge from the chosen model: you may well be left with an emotional burden following your reflections, and you need to ensure that you are equipped, mentally and physically, to deal with this.

An important consideration when choosing a model is whether or not it has a *critical* perspective. This doesn't mean that it is negative, but rather that the model espouses more than just personal introspection. In nursing practice it is important that you consider the whole practice milieu, take the viewpoints of others into consideration, consider policy/knowledge and procedures, and take action (where required) within the practice environment. This is rather more complex than simple personal reflection, but it is a requirement of the practising nurse: 'The nurse practises within a statutory framework and code of ethics delivering nursing practice (care) that is appropriately based on research, evidence and critical thinking that effectively responds to the needs of individual clients (patients) and diverse populations' (NMC 2010: 11).

Your choice of model is a personal one. There is limited direction on how to choose a model, other than to say that it should be 'appropriate'. Just as there are differences in opinion regarding definitions of reflection, there are divergent views regarding the use of models (e.g. Andresen *et al.* 2000; Rolfe *et al.* 2001). However, we recommend the use of the model proposed by Boud *et al.* (1985) as it strongly supports critical reflexivity (see also Boud and Walker 1990, 1993). This model proposes the following phases:

1   *Return* to the experience (a brief acknowledgement only, not a full description).
2   *Attend* to the feeling (make a note of how you felt).
3   *Associate* (new information resulting from reflection is associated with exisiting knowledge and attitudes).
4   *Integrate* (the same new information is integrated with exisiting knowledge).
5   *Validate* (evidence is used to test any new assumptions resulting from association and integration and ascertain whether there are any inconsistencies or contradictions).
6   *Appropriate* (take on the new knowledge as one's own).

What is useful about this approach is that when you choose specific experiences to reflect upon, your personal feelings are not a major part of the analysis, although you do *attend* to them by taking note of them and being or becoming aware of them. In this model you are asked to re-evaluate the experience, and to do so you use *association*, whereby new information from the reflection is associated with existing knowledge and attitudes and the relationships are observed. You then use *integration*, identifying the nature of the relationships that have been observed in the association phase and drawing new conclusions and insights. You then test these new assumptions by *validation* to ascertain whether there are contradictions or inconsistencies. This phase ensures that you are bringing *evidence* into your reflection, and thus your portfolio. In the final phase you *appropriate* the information from your reflection into your knowledge base for practice.

Approaches to reflection

As indicated in the previous section, we advocate models of reflection that avoid being overtly personal. Broadly speaking this means a three-phase approach (Brechin 2000):

1 Critical analysis
2 Critical reflexivity
3 Critical action

When you reflect, you need to ask yourself more than the obvious, basic questions such as: What happened? How did I feel? What would I do next time? Instead you should begin to examine the practice context – the *world* in which your practice and where your reflections took place. More importantly, you should begin to examine and provide *evidenc*e to support your claim to competence in a given area of clinical practice.

Begin your reflections by critically analysing the knowledge, theories, policy, and practice that inform the situation. This ensures that you have an informed basis upon which to perform your reflections and subsequent actions. It will also help you to recognize other people's perspectives in a given situation. Reflecting without this analysis of your knowledge-base may make your analysis uninformed, or worse, misinformed (see above). In Phase 2, you reflect on your reflections so far using your chosen model of reflection. This is reflexivity, and it provides a deeper analysis which permits you to question your personal values and assumptions. In Phase 3 you take action related to your analysis of your knowledge base and your subsequent personal reflections.

Applying reflection to your portfolio

As we discussed earlier a good approach to integrating your chosen model within your portfolio is to select one or a number of key competencies (NMC 2010) with which to work. For example, you may wish to reflect upon elements of the domain entitled 'communication and interpersonal skills', using this as a sub-theme in your portfolio. Let's look at a scenario to examine this part of the process a little further.

Scenario: Chahna

Chahna is a recently qualified general nurse. She wishes to explore the notion that her approach to communication is individualized and person-centred. She examines this using the heading 'communication and interpersonal skills' as a sub-theme for her portfolio. She decides to explain how this approach originated from her university nursing school, the philosophy of which espoused 'person-centred care'. By presenting parts of the curriculum as evidence, she suggests that this approach permeated the curriculum. She follows this up with an extract from her competence assessment documentation that shows she was deemed proficient at person-centred communication during her training.

To build upon this competence, Chahna describes evidence of how she uses person-centred communication in her current nursing practice. In her portfolio she includes philosophy statements, examples of nursing documentation and performance review information.

If you were gathering evidence, as Chahna did, you might consider collecting the following information to include in the sub-theme of 'communication and interpersonal skills':

- Your school/faculty philosophy (if you are studying at university or, if you are qualified, for the school at which you studied).
- The curriculum that underpinned your nurse education (or a synopsis of it/ the relevant parts of it).
- An extract from your competence assessment documentation that shows you were becoming proficient in this area.
- University transcript (which can usually be requested from the university, if available).
- Philosophy statements from your workplace.
- Examples of nursing documentation.
- Performance review information.
- Relevant modules, grades and related competency documents.
- Care plans.
- Personal essays.

Once you have this first sub-theme prepared (below we have suggested 'care delivery'), you can commence your reflection on the evidence. We suggest the three-phase approach outlined below.

A three-phase approach

Phase 1: critical analysis

Commencing with *critical analysis* will help you to decide which information is useful to keep, and which to discard. Examine the knowledge, theories, policy and practice that you have presented under the theme of 'care delivery'. You may be looking at, and taking abstracts from, a range of materials from personal essays and care plans to local policy and audit results. Thus, this reflection will move from your student training to your current practice in the clinical environment. This process is a continually evolving one, and you can return at any time to build upon each section.

In order to give structure to your portfolio, it is important to add *commentary* or *dialogue* to this initial phase. You could begin with a simple introduction to the sub-theme, explaining a little bit about it, and then introduce and explain each piece of evidence that you include. Make a note of:

- Why you included it
- Why it is important
- Its relevance to the sub-theme
- What you have learned from re-examining it

Phase 2: critical reflexivity

In this phase you engage in self-monitoring to given standards and norms (Brechin 2000) and a more personalized type of reflection. You could perhaps examine elements of your current role in relation to care delivery and show, using evidence, how you are capable of meeting the required standards of your area of work, or within your job description. You also need to engage in some personal introspection, *questioning personal values and assumptions*, in order to come to a *negotiated understanding*. Now a more personalized reflection can take place using the model proposed by Boud *et al.* (1985) described above.

Select specific episodes within your sub-theme that could take you to new understandings in the context of your current practice. Don't worry if these episodes, chosen because they have significance to you, appear rather random and unconnected: this is perfectly natural as life does not follow the linear, organized logic that we are attempting to apply to the portfolio. Keep a record of your reflections so that they can be organized later. Some may even relate to a *different* sub-theme on further reflection.

When choosing episodes on which to reflect you may find Benner's (2000) categorization helpful as a general guide:

- interventions that really made a difference;
- interventions that went unusually well;
- those in which there was a breakdown of some description (e.g. of communication);
- those that were ordinary and typical;
- those that captured the 'essence of nursing';
- those that were particularly demanding.

Let's look at a scenario to examine this part of the process a little further.

Scenario: Elaborating on a sub-theme

As Chahna has decided to elaborate upon the sub-theme 'communication and interpersonal skills' within her portfolio, she thinks back to one of her first client admissions after she started on the surgical ward as a newly-qualified staff nurse (returns to the experience). A long description of the event is not necessary within this model, but re-evaluation later is key in terms of what sense she can make of this experience following critical reflection. She takes note of how she was feeling, but doesn't dwell on this (attends to the feeling). She notes that she was a little nervous during the admission, but as Boud and Walker (1990) describes, having noticed these feelings she discharges them and lets them go. The feelings are now of less importance than her ultimate new learning from the event. She notes that she was more concerned about the documentation and less concerned with the patient, and therefore did not truly apply a person-centred approach.

She then realizes that she had underestimated how much using unfamiliar documentation would distract her. While she was fully prepared for the type of forms she had used during her nurse training, she had not received, nor thought to ask for, information on these new forms but as they were broadly similar to those she had used in training, she thought she would be fine. However, looking back on her previous experience of admission procedures, there seems to be more emphasis on holistic assessment of the patient than is borne out by her recent experience (association). Chahna includes the relevant documents relating to past admission procedures in her portfolio, as well as related modules from her undergraduate programme.

Chahna then does some related reading and discovers that nursing documentation, while professing to be based on a 'holistic approach' can actually still encourage nurses to use a depersonalized, medical model of care (Hyde et al. 2006). She also realizes that her knowledge base in this area (patient assessment) may need a little updating (integration). To address this she undertakes some learning in patient assessment: effective consultation and history-taking. This learning zone contains a self-assessment questionnaire which she completes. The answers are provided in the relevant journal the following week, so to provide evidence of her new learning Chahna includes her correct answers in her portfolio, as well as a reference to the Hyde article and her notes on this.

*

Through her reflections on her practice and her reading, Chahna realized that her person-centered communication could be improved during admission procedures. She improved her knowledge by reading, and also engaged a mentor in the practice area to supervise her during the next admission. She also approached her ward manager with a view to suggesting improvements to documentation (appropriation).

Phase 3: critical action

At this point you are now moving on to a key phase in the stages of the reflective process: *critical action*. Here you need to develop a sound skill base, used with awareness of context, to develop 'mutual understanding' and be able to problem-solve (Brechin 2000). Chahna's skill base in the area of assessment is already emerging through her reading. However, she may also begin to examine ways that she can follow through on her recommendations in the clinical area. Getting involved in an audit of nursing documentation could be one way to do this. Alternatively, she could seek the views of relatives via a comment box provided on the ward.

Like Chahna, you may decide that improvement of your own skills might include working alongside your supervisor during subsequent admissions, or whatever is your chosen task procedure. Even if you have been qualified for quite some time, expressing your learning needs in this way is *not* a retrograde step. Quite the reverse. This is one of the key functions of a portfolio: you hope to demonstrate achievement of individual learning goals, knowledge and skill development over time. This cannot be achieved by standing still.

For all sorts of reasons you may lack confidence with particular aspects of your nursing practice and it is best to acknowledge these deficits and aim to deal with and improve them. You must always acknowledge your own *scope of practice*, work within that and seek to improve it. In doing so you are actively engaging in the problem-solving process.

Mapping your journey

It is also important to map out your journey in the reflective process. You begin by outlining your background knowledge in the chosen sub-theme (Phase 1), followed by critical reflection on an incident (Phase 2), and finally you suggest and take action in practice (Phase 3). As mentioned above, your commentary on each phase is very important. In the final analysis, consider which original items (from Phase 1) are relevant to your final conclusions and actions in this reflective cycle, and retain *only those*. Try to weave the three phases together so that your account makes cogent sense were it to be read by another person. The following aspects should be crystal clear:

- What you are talking about
- Why you included the information you did
- What your prior learning was
- What your personal reflections/reflexivity are
- What your new learning is
- What action you took or will take in practice

You have to be selective about the material you retain. For Chahna to hold on to 25 articles on admission procedures would be unmanageable. She probably hasn't even read them all. However, her descriptions of her detailed learning in relation to the key articles she *did* read should obviously be retained in her portfolio. Remember, as we discussed in Chapter 1, sometimes with portfolio work there is a tendency to just randomly throw everything into a folder (the 'shopping trolley' approach). For a successful portfolio you *must* be disciplined and maintain a cohesive structure so that the information is easily found and consistently relevant. Such a structure will of course also make it much easier to add new information as time goes on.

With this episode of reflection complete, organized and added to the portfolio, it becomes what is known as an *entry*. Finally, you may like to asses the complete entry in terms of the following (Hull *et al.* 2005):

- Have you been honest and sincere?
- Have you been positive?
- Have you expressed yourself in a variety of ways (e.g. commentary, mind-maps etc.)?
- Have you been dilligent with regard to issues of confidentiality (see below)?

The challenges of building a reflective portfolio

There are many challenges when engaging in reflection and constructing a portfolio. The very notion of it may fill you with dread. As we have said, the best approach is to start small, begin at the very beginning and proceed from there. It is very unlikely that this task will be achieved in a day, or even two, or even more, so take your time and devote specific quiet periods to the activity. The process is time-consuming, however, once you have begun to write and develop your portfolio it will get easier and keeping it updated will be easier still.

If in the process of reflection you encounter emotional issues that have particular resonance for you and evoke negative feelings that you are unable to deal with effectively, you are advised to seek help from a professional such as a counsellor or psychologist. There should be no shame or stigma associated with seeking counselling for your emotions, as nursing can be a stressful career and you will not be alone.

There are other ways that you will need to protect yourself (and others) within the portfolio. Client confidentiality is *crucial*: you must ensure that there are no identifying features of any clients or patients discussed. Furthermore, you must treat the documents in your portfolio as you would any other documentation in your nursing practice: it could, if the situation arose, form part of a court or legal proceeding. Thus, your portfolio should not be a 'centre for catharsis' or a detailed documentation of client care, but a *selective discussion of discrete elements of your own nursing practice*.

Professional requirements

The reason for the popularity of reflection is not merely a historical legacy associated with scholarly work such as that of Schön. While it may sometimes seem to be something that is driven by the academics in nursing, there is very clear and tangible interest in reflection in nursing practice with the aim of encouraging nurses to become reflective practitioners at a professional level in the UK and elsewhere. The National Health Service Management Executive (NHSME) (1993) and United Kingdom Central Council for Nursing, Midwifery and Health Visiting (UKCC) (1997) advocate the use of reflection to support professional practice (see also Wallace 1999). Indeed, the NMC suggests that 'All nurses must be self-aware and recognise how their own values, principles and assumptions may affect their practice. They must maintain their own personal and professional development, learning from experience, through supervision, feedback, reflection and evaluation' (2010: 20). A key to achieving this outcome is the development of reflective skills and this is a requirement within the competency framework for nurses.

A portfolio is recommended by the NMC for those nurses who are involved with supporting and teaching nursing students: 'Nurses and midwives may wish to develop a portfolio of evidence ... to demonstrate how they are developing the knowledge, skills and competence related to supporting learning and assessment in practice' (2008: 15).

The NMC's guidance related to your ongoing CPD is outlined in Table 2.1. PREP requires that in order to maintain your registration as a nurse you must undertake at least 35 hours of learning activity relevant to your practice in the three years prior to re-registration and keep a record of this in your profile. Your PREP profile might be called upon by the NMC as part of their audit process. This requirement is of course in addition to the mandatory requirement of 450 hours practice in your discipline or successful undertaking of a 'back to nursing course' within the same time period. The NMC suggests that you may meet this PREP/CPD standard in many ways and there is no set formula, nor is there a need to accumulate recognized points or credits. Your portfolio will not receive official approval; hence it is very personal to you, particularly in terms of what you choose to learn and also how you choose to manage the learning that results from your reflections. However, your learning needs to be relevant to the area in which you are working, or an area in which you plan to specialize in the future. A summary of the NMC's PREP requirements is given in Table 2.2.

Table 2.1 NMC CPD guidance

- The NMC recommends that you develop a profile, which can be a component of a portfolio.
- The portfolio is not mandatory, but is a useful storage mechanism for your profile.
- Your portfolio will not receive official approval.
- Meeting this PREP/CPD standards may be achieved in many ways and there is no set formula, nor is there a need to accumulate recognized points or credits.

Table 2.2 PREP requirements

- You need to record in your profile 35 hours of learning activity relevant to your practice that has taken place in the three years prior to your next registration with the NMC.
- Your PREP profile may be called upon by the NMC as part of their audit process.
- There is a mandatory requirement of 450 hours practice in your discipline or successful undertaking of a 'back to nursing course' in the three years prior to your next registration.

In order to manage the collection and documentation of PREP as *profiles* within your portfolio, reflection can be a useful tool. Gather the relevant material and reflect upon it in the same way as has been described for a portfolio reflection in this chapter.

Pause for Thought

- Can you think of any benefits to using reflection in your practice?

Conclusion

You should now have some understanding of the background to, and meaning of, reflection in nursing. You will hopefully be able to choose a model of reflection and engage in a cycle of reflection to create a portfolio entry. You should also be aware of the challenges that reflection throws up and how to deal with these, along with the all-important issues of confidentiality and the continued registration requirements of the NMC in relation to CPD/PREP.

Summary

- Reflection has been an important concept within nursing practice and education for almost 30 years.
- Reflection has become synonymous with portfolio development in nursing.

- Reflection means looking back on events but, in the context of nursing, structured reflection using a model is the preferred method.
- Structured reflection is about learning from practice.
- Reflection is usually a personal choice (for your portfolio).
- When using a reflective model it is important to carry out *all* the required steps.
- Always remember to maintain patient confidentiality.

References

Andresen, L., Boud, D. and Cohen, R. (2000) Experience-based learning, in G. Foley (ed.) *Understanding Adult Education and Training*. Sydney: Allen & Unwin.

Benner, P.D. (2000) *From Novice to Expert: Excellence and Power in Clinical Nursing Practice*. Harlow: Prentice Hall.

Boud, D. *et al.* (1985) Promoting reflection in learning: a model, in D. Boud, D. Walker and R. Keogh, *Reflection: Turning Experience into Learning*. London: Kogan Page.

Boud, D. and Walker, D. (1990) Making the most of experience, *Studies in Continuing Education*, 12(2): 62–80.

Boud, D. and Walker, D. (1993) Barriers to reflection on experience, in D. Boud, R. Cohen and D. Walker, *Using Experience For Learning*. Buckingham: SRHE/ Open University Press.

Brechin, A. (2000) Introducing critical practice, in A. Brechin, H. Brown and E.M. London, *Critical Practice in Health and Social Care*. London: Sage.

Duffy, A. (2008) Guided reflection: a discussion of the essential components, *British Journal of Nursing*, 17(5): 334–9.

Gibbs, G. (1988) *Learning by Doing: A Guide to Teaching and Learning Methods*. Oxford: Oxford Brookes University.

Hull, C., Redfern, J. and Shuttleworth, A. (2005) *Profiles and Portfolios: A Guide for Health & Social Care*. Basingstoke: Palgrave Macmillan.

Hyde, A. *et al.* (2006) Social regulation, medicalisation and the nurse's role: insights from an analysis of nursing documentation, *International Journal of Nursing Studies*, 43(6): 735–44.

McMullan, M. *et al.* (2003) Portfolios and assessment of competence: a review of the literature, *Journal of Advanced Nursing*, 41: 283–94.

NHSME (National Health Service Management Executive) (1993) *A Vision For the Future*. London: Department of Health.

NMC (Nursing and Midwifery Council) (2006) *The PREP Handbook*. London: NMC.

NMC (Nursing and Midwifery Council) (2008) *Standards to Support Learning and Assessment in Practice*, 2nd edn. London: NMC.

NMC (Nursing and Midwifery Council) (2010) *Standards for Pre-registration Nursing Education*. London: NMC.

Rolfe, G., Freshwater, D. and Jasper, M. (2001) *Critical Reflection for Nursing and the Helping Professions: A User's Guide*. Baskingstoke: Palgrave.

Schön, D.A. (1983) *The Reflective Practitioner*. New York: Basic Books.

UKCC (United Kingdom Central Council for Nursing, Midwifery and Health Visiting) (1997) *PREP and You*. London: UKCC.

Wallace, M. (1999) *Life-Long Learning: PREP in Action*. Oxford: Churchill Livingstone.

What should your portfolio look like?

3

By the end of this chapter you will:

○ Be able to take the first steps in creating your portfolio.
○ Know how to seek assistance with your portfolio.
○ Understand more about the shape and content of your portfolio.
○ Understand how your CV fits with your portfolio.
○ Understand how to link portfolio entries together to develop the structure.
○ Be able to show evidence of your competence in your portfolio.

In this chapter we will begin to explore what your portfolio might look like, and what you might expect it to contain. The chapter explains the basic requirements for portfolio development, and shows you how a portfolio actually develops.

What your portfolio looks like is actually a matter of personal preference. Hence, you should choose a format that suits you best. The more traditional form of portfolio has been a ring binder, which makes use of tabbed dividers and plastic page-holders to keep things neat. However, ring-binder portfolios can cause problems with storage and confidentiality. Often when nurses wish to take their portfolio to work with them there is nowhere to store it safely, under lock and key. Ring binders also have a tendency to fall apart, usually at the worst possible moment. So, if you choose a ring binder you need to make sure that it is strong and replace it when it begins to wear out. You also need to consider where you are going to store it, both at home and at work, and how you will transport it, should you need to. Unfortunately, this type of port-folio is not something that will neatly fit into a handbag or satchel, especially if you have developed it over time, so a good strong bag is needed as well.

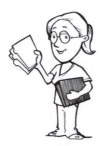

Even though there are drawbacks to using a ring binder to store your portfolio, it can nevertheless be very effective and does not require any specialist knowledge, as an e-portfolio does. If you choose this type of portfolio arrangement:

- Use a strong ring binder
- Use tabbed dividers
- Use plastic page-holders
- Keep things neat
- Store your portfolio safely and securely

It is also important to have clear signposts throughout your portfolio so that both you and other readers can find their way around easily. The organization of your portfolio is discussed throughout this chapter.

Remember!

Your portfolio needs structure: a beginning, a middle and an 'end'.

First steps

To help you begin, and avoid the dangers of procrastination (often borne out of fear) remember the first three steps towards getting started, listed in Chapter 1 (see p. 9): 1) Decide, 2) Commit, 3) Explore

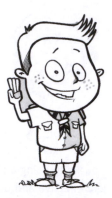

Deciding to start your portfolio is the first step. If you have got this far you are doing well. *Commit* yourself by promising to complete this task, but also by taking small steps (allocate some time to getting started and keep to it). Be warned: as part of your *exploration* you may come across examples of other portfolios, perhaps from study days or courses, or from observing undergraduate nursing students. While in some ways these sample portfolios can be helpful, they may also be misleading as student or postgraduate nurses often use their portfolios for very different purposes than you. In fact, using an 'educational' portfolio as an example to follow might cause you more confusion and put you off as a consequence. By the same token, if you developed your own portfolio as a nursing student, you may well find that it does not fit your current purpose, now that you are qualified. Equally, your original undergraduate portfolio may have been useful at the time, but it has been left to stagnate over the last year or two. As you progress through your nursing career your values, beliefs and philosophy towards your practice often change as you advance in your nursing experience. This is why we say that creating and maintaining a portfolio is a *journey* rather than a *destination*.

So, it is best to start afresh. None of your previous work will go to waste and can easily be drawn into the new portfolio if it is relevant. Remember, the portfolio is a very personal piece of work; therefore there are no right and wrong ways to compile a new one.

The fourth step is *identify*:

Identify: pinpoint the approach that works best for you, along with potential barriers to success. Consider how you will overcome such barriers.

You will have examined your learning style in Chapter 1 (see Table 1.1), and this will help you to identify what type of approach to learning you prefer to take when beginning your portfolio.

Pause for Thought

- What type of learner are you?

- What approach is best for you?

- Are there challenges to getting started or compiling your portfolio?

- How can you seek to overcome these challenges?

Seeking assistance

Step 5 is:

> *Negotiate:* group discussions and reflection are very useful. Discuss your thoughts and decisions so far with colleagues and your reflective friend. Always be open to ideas and suggestions others make for improvement.

One challenge you may encounter relates to asking for help. Remember, students who are completing portfolios often have the guidance of tutors, preceptors or reflective friends to help them develop their portfolio and guide them through the work. Sometimes, however, as a qualified staff nurse you can feel a little bit at sea without such mentors. As outlined in Chapter 1, try to identify someone who will be willing to act as your reflective friend – someone you can bounce ideas off, share your concerns with and who will help you with your reflections. You should also consider group work.

When sharing your developmental ideas with others there are one or two things you need to keep in mind. Firstly, as mentioned above, *confidentiality is paramount*, so you will need to ensure that when sharing your work it will not be used (or abused) by others. Secondly, have confidence, and encourage confidence in your readers. Very often people say, 'Oh I'm not an expert'; 'I wouldn't know anything about that', but this may be because they haven't used a portfolio before, or don't have the relevant qualifications. This does not mean that they will be unable to offer constructive feedback, nor that they have to be, necessarily, an expert in the field. You may well find yourself seeking a lay opinion from a friend as well as professional views from your designated reflective friend.

When requesting feedback it is important to structure it by imposing (gently) deadlines for the feedback and providing some guidance about what you expect from your reader. For many elements of your portfolio you are simply seeking an opinion on the overall impression of the content on that person (be they a lay person or a fellow health professional). Ask your reader to comment on the following:

Is the portfolio . . .

- *A collection?* In other words, is there a *range* of material included?
- *Organized?* Can your critical reader navigate their way around easily? Can they suggest improvements for navigation?
- *Neat?* Does it appear untidy or difficult to follow? Is it pleasing to the eye? Could the presentation be improved in any way?
- *A cohesive account?* Is it clear? Is it obvious what the portfolio is trying to portray? Does it make sense?
- *Succinct?* Is there (in their opinion) too little or too much included? What else would they suggest you could include? What could you leave out?
- *Relevant?* Is everything (in their opinion) relevant?

Does the portfolio contain . . .

- Descriptions/outlines of work-based learning?
- Relevant evidence?
- Evidence of achievement of professional competence or learning outcomes?
- Evidence of knowledge development?

Remember you are only asking colleagues/friends to comment on the 'face validity', or the general appearance, of your portfolio, *not* the in-depth content. The content will be for you to decide, as ultimately the portfolio is about you and your nursing practice. 'Face validity' is about whether, on the face of it (at a glance) the portfolio appears to be what it says it is. You are asking people to comment on whether the portfolio appears to be:

- a collection;
- a cohesive account;

and whether or not it contains:

- work-based learning;
- relevant evidence;
- evidence of achievement of professional competence.

Pause for Thought

- Consider what benefit you think a lay reader might be to you.

- Consider who you might like to be your lay reader.

- Are there any drawbacks to having a lay reader?

- How can you address and rectify these drawbacks?

In order to ensure your portfolio reaches these standards, you need to consider the next step, *planning*.

The shape and content of your portfolio

Step 6 is:

> *Plan:* now plan your strategy based on *realistic targets.*

Your portfolio should have an integrated, cohesive approach. By this we mean that the whole document is signposted throughout, so that the way it all fits together is clear. Begin the portfolio with an introduction. Here you should define the purpose of your portfolio and provide a preliminary outline of what readers can expect. An example is given in Figure 3.1. The introduction is then followed by a table of contents (see Figure 3.2). In ring binder form, this will be a simple list, however in an e-portfolio the list may also provide instant links to each section.

Each section of the portfolio as it relates to the contents page should have its own tabbed divider within the ring binder, with the name of the section written on it. With an e-portfolio each section could have its own electronic file.

My portfolio

Name:	Anna Tokarev
Grade:	E
Area of work:	Orthopaedic nursing

Introduction

Photo

A portfolio is a collection and cohesive account of work-based learning that contains relevant evidence from practice and critical reflection on this evidence (Timmins 2008). The aim of this portfolio is to provide evidence of my ongoing competence, maintenance and development in the following areas:

1 Professional values

2 Communication and interpersonal skills

3 Nursing practice and decision-making

4 Leadership, management and team working

Using these competency domains as subheadings, I will analyse and explain my ongoing learning and competence development in each domain. To do this I will select episodes of work-based learning, and other evidence of learning in order to demonstrate proficiency. A model of reflection (state) is used to further analyse these experiences, draw out beneficial learning and identify further learning needs.

The portfolio is divided into seven sections. The first section comprises my CV, followed by five subsections. The final section summarizes the learning to date. Specific learning episodes within these sections are listed in the Contents on the next page.

Figure 3.1 Example of an introduction to a portfolio.

	Page
Introduction	
Section 1: *CV*	
Section 2: *Summary of ongoing nursing experience*	
Section 3: *Professional values*	
Introduction	
Key elements from my undergraduate programme	
Working with older people in orthopaedic nursing	
Reflection: aspects of the Code of Conduct – *confidentiality*	
Courses attended	
Conclusion	
Summary of learning and identified learning needs: where do I go from here?	
Section 4: *Communication and interpersonal skills*	
Introduction	
My philosophy of care	
Case study: communicating with older people – *total hip replacement*	
Reflection: person-centred communication – *postoperative care*	
Conclusion	
Summary of learning and identified learning needs: where do I go from here?	

Section 5 : _Nursing practice and decision-making_	
Introduction	
Examples of documentation from the ward (2010–11)	
Testimonies from other staff	
Courses attended	
Reflection: decision-making – _contacting the doctor on call during night duty_	
Conclusion	
Summary of learning and identified learning needs: where do I go from here?	
Section 6 : _Leadership, management and team working_	
Introduction	
Outline of management modules from undergraduate course	
Essay on ward management completed during undergraduate course	
Testimonies from other staff	
Reflection 1: learning during undergraduate course – _where does it fit in now?_	
Reflection 2: working with my supervisor – _managing the ward_	
Conclusion	
Summary of learning and identified learning needs: where do I go from here?	
Section 7: _Summary_	

Figure 3.2 Example of portfolio contents page.

Including your CV

Including a specific CV within your portfolio for employment-seeking purposes is helpful. It has been found that employers prefer to refer to and use candidates' CVs rather than their portfolios (Patrick-Williams and Bennett 2010). It is not clear why employers choose this option, but it could be due to the lengthy (and sometimes unwieldy) nature of some portfolios, which would take too much time to read and assimilate. In addition, a lack of consistency of format may make comparison between candidates too difficult. In some cases the portfolio may lack the specifics required for the application.

So, to be on the safe side, always include a CV as part of your portfolio. The CV is in any case a useful summary of your overall nursing experience and educational achievements and therefore represents an easily accessible record to guide your portfolio development.

An example of a 'portfolio CV' is provided in Figure 3.3. As your CV grows it can incorporate other sections such as 'publications', 'public honours', 'oral presentations', along with further educational study you have undertaken since qualifying, attendance at conferences, study days and short courses, committee membership and voluntary work.

Within the portfolio your CV could be followed by a summary of your ongoing nursing experiences which would provide more detail than merely dates of employment and role. It is very important to include a record of hours worked in practice, as you will need this for your PREP requirements. Table 3.1 is an example of how you could record your clinical practice hours. However, the choice is entirely yours. Note that only a brief synopsis is provided under the heading 'specific experiences'. This can be expanded to include more detail, for example, about the ward (e.g. patient numbers, conditions) and other specific information such as specialist/generic skills required and even types of equipment used, particularly if you are working in a specialized practice area such as coronary care, intensive care or accident and emergency (A&E).

Curriculum vitae

NAME: Ms Anna Tokarev

ADDRESS: 21 The Heath

                         Binkely upon Thames

                         London

                         W12 32C

TELEPHONE: 09477 359 028

DATE OF BIRTH: 3 August 1988

Educational programmes and professional awards

Sept 2006–Sept 2009   **Abraham Franklin School of Nursing**

                                University of Bedwickham, England

Registration: Registered general nurse (NMC)

Degree: Bachelor of Nursing Science (2:1 Hons)

Professional employment record

Sept 2009–April 2010   Staff nurse, surgical ward

                                Bington Hospital, Bington, Surrey, England

April 2010–present   Staff nurse, orthopaedic ward, St Cecelia's Hospital,

                                Bedwickham

Figure 3.3 Example of a basic CV for a portfolio.

Table 3.1 Record of hours worked in practice

Dates	Role	Hours in practice	Specific experiences	Related competencies	Portfolio examples
September 2009– April 2010	Staff nurse, surgical ward	1,120 hours	Pre-operative and post-operative care of patients following orthopaedic surgery	Developing professional and ethical practice Care delivery Care management Personal and professional development	See Section 3 See Section 4
April 2010– present	Staff nurse, ortho-paedic ward	750 hours	Pre-operative and post-operative care of patients following orthopaedic surgery	Developing professional and ethical practice Care delivery Care management Personal and professional development	See Section 5 See Section 6

Linking your entries together

You will now see that you can link your clinical experience to chosen competence headings to demonstrate where your clinical practice hours link into your portfolio. You then 'signpost' your experiences to the specific competencies that you have included in the portfolio. A weakness of nursing portfolios is their failure to link the various 'artefacts' together. Remember, in your nursing practice you function as an *integrated whole*. All your work-based professional knowledge, your studies, reading and additional courses should come together as one, demonstrating to others the 'Professional You'.

The basic structure of your portfolio should now begin to emerge and you can begin to examine your previous and current nursing practice and collect items ('artefacts') that relate to specific competencies on which you wish to reflect and/or that you hope to develop. This is the point where you can begin to use the domains of competence to help structure your portfolio and your thinking.

Developing the structure

Your planning should include thinking about ways you can keep the artefacts and entries organized within your portfolio. This means finding an overarching framework that can both contain and direct your writing, evidence, inserts and reflections. This framework draws your work together in a cohesive way and guards against the 'shopping trolley' approach, which apart from being disorganized and difficult to navigate, fails to demonstrate any real purpose or meaning to your portfolio. In Chapter 2 we suggested using the following as over-arching frameworks to structure your portfolio:

- domains of competence;
- a model of reflection.

Both serve to give the portfolio structure. As a reminder, the four broad domains of competence (NMC 2010) are:

- professional values;
- communication and interpersonal skills;
- nursing practice and decision-making;
- leadership, management and team working.

In the Republic of Ireland there are five domains (An Bord Altranais 2004):

- professional/ethical practice;
- holistic approaches to care and the integration of knowledge;
- interpersonal relationships;
- organization and management of care;
- personal and professional development.

Similarly, if you are working in specific nursing roles such as nurse manager, nurse consultant, advanced nurse practitioner or specialist nurse, there may be specific domains of competence or proficiencies relevant to your role that you might choose to help you organize your portfolio. For example, in the Republic of Ireland the key competencies for advanced nurse practitioner are outlined by the An Bord Altranais (2004) as follows:

- autonomy in clinical practice;
- pioneering professional and clinical leadership;
- expert practitioner;
- researcher.

These would serve as useful and relevant subheadings to provide structure to your portfolio if you are working in this type of role. Any categories relevant to your area, discipline or practice may be used. The choice is yours: there are no hard and fast rules about choosing relevant competencies to guide your professional development. However, you should give careful thought to your choice of competency and be able to simply explain in your portfolio where your choice of approach emerged from.

Your chosen headings now form the individual sections of your portfolio.

Remember!

Choose suitable subheadings (sections) to begin to organize your portfolio.

Implementation

Step 7 is:

Implement: begin to implement your strategy in a disciplined manner.

If you choose to use the NMC (2010) domains of competence as sections within your portfolio, your plan will look something like that shown in Figure 3.4.

Introduction

Table of contents

CV

Section 1: Professional values

Section 2: Communication and interpersonal skills

Section 3: Nursing practice and decision-making

Section 4: Leadership, management and team working

Figure 3.4 Putting the plan into practice: your portfolio sections.

As it stands this basic structure for Figure 3.4 appears too sparse and may lead to the 'shopping trolley' approach. The answer is to add subheadings to create subsections. More detailed information about the domains you have chosen can be found in *Standards for Pre-registration Nursing Education* (NMC 2010). This document outlines the broad standards (*generic competencies*) required for each domain. For example, the generic standard for 'communication and interpersonal skills' is:

> All nurses must use excellent communication and interpersonal skills. Their communications must always be safe, effective, compassionate and respectful. They must communicate effectively using a wide range of strategies and interventions including the effective use of communication technologies. Where people have a disability nurses must be able to work with service users and others to obtain the information needed to make reasonable adjustments that promote optimum health and enable equal access to services.
>
> (NMC 2010: 15)

Within the domains of competence you will also find examples of *field competencies* that specifically apply within each domain and within each discipline of nursing. Field competencies provide very detailed descriptions of the types of knowledge, behaviours and skills you are required to demonstrate as evidence of achieving competence within the given domain. This level of detail, if applied to your portfolio, will provide room for more in-depth discussion and presentation of evidence (artefacts, entries, reflections). For example, in relation to the competence 'communication and interpersonal skills' for adult nurses there is one over-arching *field competence* and eight further, more detailed, *field competencies* (NMC 2010) (see Figure 3.5).

When you are putting together your portfolio you need to:

1 Select the competence domain (e.g. 'communication and interpersonal skills')

and then . . .

2 Select the generic competence and field competencies that apply.

Communication and interpersonal skills

Overarching field competence

Adult nurses must demonstrate the ability to listen with empathy. They must be able to respond warmly and positively to people of all ages who may be anxious, distressed, or facing problems with their health and wellbeing.

Field competencies

1   All nurses must build partnerships and therapeutic relationships through safe, effective and non-discriminatory communication. They must take account of individual differences, capabilities and needs.

2   All nurses must use a range of communication skills and technologies to support person-centred care and enhance quality and safety. They must ensure people receive all the information they need in a language and manner that allows them to make informed choices and share decision-making. They must recognise when language interpretation or other communication support is needed and know how to obtain it.

3   All nurses must use the full range of communication methods, including verbal, non-verbal and written, to acquire, interpret and record their knowledge and understanding of people's needs. They must be aware of their own values and beliefs and the impact this may have on their communication with others. They must take account of the many different ways in which people communicate and how these may be influenced by ill health, disability and other factors, and be able to recognise and respond effectively when a person finds it hard to communicate.

3.1   *__Adult nurses__ must promote the concept, knowledge and practice of self-care with people with acute and long-term conditions, using a range of communication skills and strategies.*

4   All nurses must recognise when people are anxious or in distress and respond effectively, using therapeutic principles, to promote their wellbeing, manage personal safety and resolve conflict. They must use effective communication strategies and negotiation techniques to achieve best outcomes, respecting the dignity and human rights of all concerned. They must know when to consult a third party and how to make referrals for advocacy, mediation or arbitration.

5   All nurses must use therapeutic principles to engage, maintain and, where appropriate, disengage from professional caring relationships, and must always respect professional boundaries.

6   All nurses must take every opportunity to encourage health-promoting behaviour through education, role modelling and effective communication.

7   All nurses must maintain accurate, clear and complete records, including the use of electronic formats, using appropriate and plain language.

8   All nurses must respect individual rights to confidentiality and keep information secure and confidential in accordance with the law and relevant ethical and regulatory frameworks, taking account of local protocols. They must also actively share personal information with others.

Figure 3.5 Field competencies related to domain: communication and interpersonal skills (NMC 2010:15).

Now outline the competence domain as one of your main portfolio sections, describing the generic competence at the beginning. Then describe the overarching field competencies and list the other field competencies as your subsections (see Figure 3.6). This process should help to guide the selection of evidence that will ultimately support the conclusion that you are competent in this particular area of your nursing practice. It can also be helpful to use the language within the selected competence to structure your introduction to each subsection.

The next stage is to use your chosen model of reflection to 'unpack' your chosen domain standard, thus enabling you to examine your knowledge base within that area.

Section 2: communication and interpersonal skills	➤ Adult nurses must demonstrate the ability to listen with empathy. They must be able to respond warmly and positively to people of all ages who may be anxious, distressed, or facing problems with their health and well-being.	
Generic competence		1 Build partnerships and therapeutic relationships.
All nurses must use excellent communication and interpersonal skills. Their communications must always be safe, effective compassionate and respectful. They must communicate effectively using a wide range of strategies and interventions including the effective use of communication technologies. Where people have a disability nurses must be able to work with service users and others to obtain the information needed to make reasonable adjustments that promote optimum health and enable equal access to services		2 Use a range of communication skills and technologies.
		3 Use the full range of communication methods.
		a *promote the concept, knowledge and practice of self-care.*
		4 Recognize when people are anxious or in distress and respond effectively.
		5 Use therapeutic principles to engage, maintain and, where appropriate, disengage from professional caring relationships.
		6 Take every opportunity to encourage health-promoting behaviour.
		7 Maintain accurate, clear and complete records.
		8 Respect individual rights to confidentiality and keep information secure.

Figure 3.6 Putting the plan into practice: your portfolio sections.

> **Remember!**
>
> Your portfolio will be easier to organize and easier to read if you include sections and subsections. Choose a method that suits you best.

Profiles

A word at this stage about profiles. Remember it is a *profile* that may be required by the NMC for audit purposes. A profile is a selection of evidence that can be extracted from your portfolio. As you build your portfolio, give some thought to which elements of it might usefully form the much simpler, and shorter, profile document. Figure 3.7 gives an example of how a profile can be created from a single portfolio entry.

Showing evidence of your competence

As a qualified nurse you will already have satisfied the NMC that you have achieved the required competencies upon registration. However, it is useful to revisit them within your portfolio, as evidence of your continued competence and lifelong learning commitment.

Your choice of portfolio sections and subsections will guide your selection of artefacts to include as evidence of your competence. It is important that whatever material you include serves as *evidence* of your competence and learning within that particular domain. The interpretation of evidence in practice moves from a mere collection of artefacts to their cohesive construction and presentation, including your reflection on the evidence presented. For example, what evidence do you have that you are 'building partnerships and therapeutic relationships'? By using the reflective framework outlined in Chapter 2 you might ask *how you came to know what you know* about 'communication and interpersonal skills'. Remember that Phase 1 of reflection is *critical analysis* (see Chapter 2, pp. 39–40). By critically analysing your nursing practice you are fulfilling a crucial task within your

Section 4: Communication and interpersonal skills	
Subsection 4.1	
Field competence: building partnerships and therapeutic relationships	
Introduction	
My philosophy of care	
Ward philosophy of care/policy and my personal commentary on this	
Case study: communicating with older people – *total hip replacement*	
Reflection: person-centred communication – *post-operative care*	
Reflection: new reflections on and understanding of essay on communication from undergraduate programme	
Evidence of hours of nursing practice	
Course/study day attendance and certificate: *developing good nurse–patient relationships*	
Testimony from patients: 'thank you' letter	
Conclusion	
Summary of learning and identified learning needs: where do I go from here?	

Figure 3.7 Example outline of a portfolio subsection that could be presented as a profile.

portfolio: critically reflecting on the evidence you have presented. Note that in Figure 3.7 reflection is carried out on both clinical practice (carrying out postoperative care) and on an academic essay (demonstrating new understandings).

Ask yourself what knowledge, theories, policies, guidelines and procedures influence and inform your competence in this domain. To answer this you may choose to include an example of course material from your nurse education programme, perhaps reflecting once again on an essay that you wrote or module descriptors related to this area of practice. You may also explore your current awareness through a description of current policies that relate to your area of practice.

Phase two of the reflective process is *critical reflexivity*, for which you should use your chosen model of reflection, critically reflecting on the evidence you have presented.

Remember!

The evidence presented needs to be relevant to the domain.

Each section and subsection in your portfolio should have a mini-introduction explaining your aims. A couple of paragraphs is usually sufficient for these. Remember, try to use the language that is specific to the chosen competence to structure your mini-introductions. For example, Anna's intro-duction to her 'communication and interpersonal skills' section is shown in Figure 3.8.

Phase three of the reflective process is *critical action*. Here you need to summarize your learning within the domain and identify future learning needs for yourself. You also need to identify actions that will address those learning needs. If, for example, you need to update your communication skills you may decide to complete some self-learning or attend a study session on the topic. Where personal learning needs exist, it is often helpful to use 'pathways' to assist you with your critical action. Table 3.2 provides four pathways to guide you towards identifying your future learning needs within any specified domain.

Using this framework, identify your personal learning needs within the section or subsection of your portfolio relating to maintaining or improving upon the specified domain of competence.

At the end of each section you should include a short summary identifying your learning needs arising from the process of reflection outlined above. You can update your entry as you gain the specific learning experiences required.

Communication and interpersonal skills

Introduction

Communication is a very important skill in nursing. Although we communicate from birth, I learnt most about communication during my nurse training. I learnt that it is really important for nurses to have good listening skills when caring for patients and their families. It is also important that we show respect at all times. A wide range of skills are used to be a good communicator and I built these up during my time as a student nurse. Above all the nurse must always be 'safe, effective compassionate and respectful' and of course we have a very important health promotion role.

Increased communication technologies are coming into play in nursing practice today, and as a nurse I need to be able to use these effectively. Within the domain of 'communication and interpersonal skills' I am going to take a close look at my skills in this area to see how I am doing now that I have been qualified for a little while. I am going to choose two particular field competencies ('building partnerships and therapeutic relationships' and 'recognizing when people are anxious or in distress, and responding effectively' to focus on and show evidence of my developing competence in communication and interpersonal skills in orthopaedic nursing practice.

Figure 3.8 Anna's introduction to the 'communication and interpersonal skills' section of her portfolio.

Table 3.2 Four pathways to identifying and planning your learning needs

Pathway	Question
Assessment of needs	What do I need to know?
Formulation of objectives	What do I need to get out of this learning?
The design of learning experiences	What type of learning experience(s) would facilitate me gaining the knowledge that I need?
Evaluation	How effective was the learning experience(s) in facilitating me gaining the knowledge and skills that I needed?

This summary section will help you with Step 8:

> *Re-examine:* as you progress, periodically question and examine your personal attitudes and values.

By outlining your learning and establishing your needs in a particular domain you are showing that you can question and appraise not only your own knowledge and skills, but your underlying attitudes and values. Remember the final phase in getting started is *persistence*. Now that you have started your portfolio you need to summon the energy to keep going. Don't give up!

Conclusion

You should now be fully equipped to make a proper start on your portfolio.

Summary

- Start now!
- Your portfolio will be easier to organize and easier to read if you divide it into sections.
- Use a format you are comfortable with – ringbinder or e-portfolio. Often simplest works best.
- Choose a portfolio framework to organize your learning and achievements. Use this framework to title your subsections (see the mind-map in Chapter one, p. 7, as a guide).
- Choose a model for reflection and identify specific elements of your experience, related to your clinical competence, to reflect upon.
- Keep a coherent flow within your portfolio and signpost as much as possible.
- Keep going!

Follow the steps, get help from others, don't procrastinate, and you will be well on your way.

References

An Bord Altranais (2004) *Requirements and Standards for Nurse Registration Education Programmes*. Dublin: An Bord Altranais.

NMC (Nursing and Midwifery Council) (2010) *Standards for Pre-registration Nursing Education*. London: NMC.

Patrick-Williams, I. and Bennett, R. (2010) The effectiveness of the professional portfolio in the hiring process of the associate degree nurse, *Teaching and Learning in Nursing*, 5(1): 44–8.

Organizing your portfolio

4

By the end of this chapter you will:

○ Appreciate the benefits of being organized.
○ Be able to choose your approach in relation to the 'portfolio hierarchy'.
○ Understand how to document practice as evidence.
○ Begin to make sense of your portfolio.

In this chapter we will explore some of the finer points of organizing your nursing portfolio. As discussed in Chapter 3, putting a structure to your portfolio, for example by using the NMC (2010) nursing competencies, will assist you in easily finding and storing items in the relevant sections and subsections. However, selecting sections and subsections within an over-arching framework is only one aspect of organizing your portfolio.

Being organized

Within your profile you need to be *orderly* in terms of your:

● information-seeking;
● information retrieval;
● information collection;
● reflections;
● writing;
● storage and filing;
● presentation.

From the outset you need to use your time efficiently and manage it effectively. Rather than randomly collecting or seeking out information for your portfolio, set aside one or two hours per week as 'portfolio time'. If you do not do this you will spend a lot of time thinking about what you *should* be doing, but doing very little. Portfolio development then becomes a stressful activity and is ultimately likely to fail.

> ## Remember!
>
> Set aside specific time each week to work on your portfolio (at least one or two hours per week).

Using set times will enable you, for example, to read an article or carry out a reflection with some level of concentration, rather than superficially attacking such tasks while you are 'on the move'. One to two hours of detailed reading, reflecting and learning is much more valuable than a sporadic collection of numerous artefacts. Planning for 'depth of learning' is also efficient behaviour. *Plan* what you are going to learn about, and stay focused within that plan. As ever, it is all about a methodical, step-by-step approach to building your portfolio over time.

Planning your time

Using an example from Chapter 3, Table 4.1 shows how you might plan your time when developing a subsection within your portfolio by outlining a sample timeline.

You will notice all the while when you are developing your portfolio that you are gathering relevant material (artefacts). For the most part this should be as methodical as possible – that is, confined to the time you have set aside for your portfolio work, and linked specifically to the domain you are working on. However, occasionally you will come across something interesting but not strictly relevant to your chosen domain at that time. It might be a newspaper article, a newly-published journal article or an unexpected 'thank

Table 4.1 A sample timeline

Week	Subject	Plan
1	**Section 4:** *Communication and interpersonal skills*	Read NMC competency
2	*Subsection 4.1*	Plan sections and subsections, outline titles
3	**Field competence: building partnerships and therapeutic relationships**	Read more about this domain
4	Introduction	Outline a brief introduction
5	My philosophy of care	Get ward philosophy/write my philosophy
6	Ward philosophy of care/policy and my personal commentary on this	Write commentary on ward philosophy
7	Case study: communicating with older people – *total hip replacement*	Write out case study
8	**Reflection:** person-centred communication – *post-operative care*	Write out reflection
9	**Reflection:** new reflections on and understanding of essay on communication from undergraduate programme	Write out reflection
10	Evidence of hours of nursing practice	Document hours worked
11	Course/study day attendance and certificate – *developing good nurse–patient relationships*	Attend study day/collect and collate information
12	Testimony from patients: 'thank you' letter	Find other evidence
13	Conclusion	Write conclusion
14	Summary of learning and identified learning needs: where do I go from here?	Summarize this subsection and revise introduction

you' letter from a patient, so you need to be organized enough to expect and deal with the unexpected. An effective approach here is to file artefacts and evidence in a 'holding area' such as a box file or an electronic folder on your computer. In this way you can keep your organized portfolio separate from your ongoing collection of material. Remember: you may not use all that you collect, and you must be selective in your choice of artefacts and evidence, depending on your portfolio's structure.

> ## Remember!
>
> Create a separate 'holding area' for new material, yet to be assigned (or not) to your main portfolio.

The shopping trolley

If you don't impose a formal structure on your portfolio, it will function simply as a receptacle, no different to your 'holding area'. As a result it will grow to an unmanageable size as your career progresses and it won't make any sense when you revisit it. You will have what we have already referred to as a 'shopping trolley' portfolio full of unrelated artefacts (see Figure 4.1).

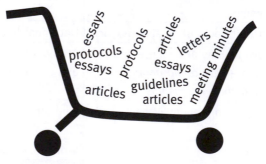

Figure 4.1 The shopping trolley.

Source: Endacott *et al.* (2004) © Elsevier, reprinted with permission

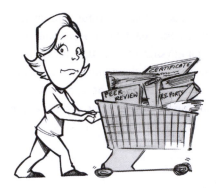

Although there are sometimes conflicting opinions about what constitutes a portfolio, there is no doubt about the fact that your evidence and reflections on your clinical practice must fit together *logically*. But how do you achieve this?

A logical structure

Having a well organized portfolio and keeping it up to date will encourage you to *use* the information, and more importantly, you will *want* to use it and be proud of it. Basic organization is discussed in Chapter 3, where the

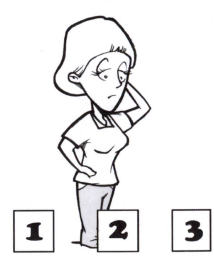

importance of subheadings and subsections was explained. Your choice will depend on many things, not least your area and level of practice. At the basic level you are well advised to structure your portfolio around the NMC competencies. However, an advanced nurse practitioner is likely to choose subheadings like 'autonomy in clinical practice', 'pioneering leadership', 'the expert practitioner' or 'the role of the researcher'. A clinical nurse specialist, on the other hand, might focus on 'clinical skills', 'patient advocacy', 'education and training' or 'audits and research'

The toast rack

Choosing a framework that provides headings for dividing your portfolio into sections allows you to move beyond the 'shopping trolley' approach. In the 'hierarchy of portfolios' (Endacott *et al.* 2004) applying this framework results in the 'toast rack' approach, where discrete subsections are used but there is usually little integration between them (see Figure 4.2).

When you file your artefacts, evidence and reflections in this way (without the introductions and summaries suggested in Chapter 3), the sections and subsections stand alone, without linking to one another. While there is nothing essentially wrong with this, it does mean that you could do a lot of work in organizing your portfolio but its impact (on the reader) will not be much greater than if you had adopted the 'shopping trolley' approach. What

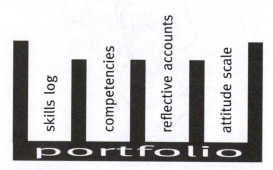

Figure 4.2 The toast rack.

Source: Endacott *et al.* (2004) © Elsevier, reprinted with permission

you need is to achieve *cohesiveness*, which leads us to consider the 'spinal column' approach.

The spinal column

Cohesiveness is about adding *dialogue* (commentary) to your portfolio: *explaining* to the reader, and to yourself, where you are going with your ideas and presentation. Using an introduction and table of contents as we discussed in Chapter 3 is the first step in attempting to integrate your work. Other ways of doing this are by providing clear signposts throughout, and adding sentences of dialogue between sections, subsections and the evidence presented. Sometimes all you need is one or two sentences, or a map outlining where everything fits within your portfolio. If you are able to do this, and provide at least some linkage, you are already moving up the hierarchy to the next level: the 'spinal column' (see Figure 4.3). This is the level of integration that we hope you will aim for when preparing your portfolio.

The 'spinal column' approach can be achieved by appropriate selection of sections and subsections. For example, if you categorize your learning

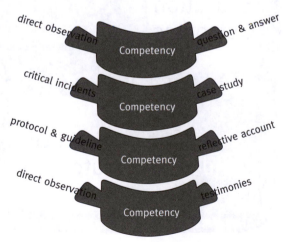

Figure 4.3 The spinal column.

Source: Endacott *et al.* (2004) © Elsevier, reprinted with permission

according to years of practice, you will have to think of ways of linking each year's learning to the next. This approach inevitably provides more structure and cohesion than either the 'shopping trolley' or 'toast rack' models. A 'layered effect' is also achieved, whereby although all the sections do not necessarily link directly to each other in an obvious way, each 'disc' of the 'backbone' builds on the previous one and supports the next. The 'spinal column' is a strong model to follow, but as time goes by you may want to take things one step further, which leads us to the next level in the hierarchy: the 'cake mix'.

The cake mix

The highest level in the portfolio hierarchy is the 'cake mix' (see Figure 4.4). To achieve this, you will need to add a descriptive dialogue (commentary) *throughout* your portfolio, taking the reader from the introduction, step-by-step

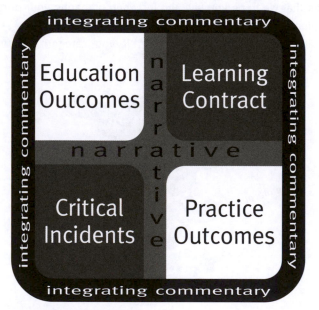

Figure 4.4 The cake mix.

Source: Endacott *et al.* (2004) © Elsevier, reprinted with permission

through the sections of the portfolio (which in the case of Figure 4.4 are 'education outcomes', 'learning contract', 'critical incidents' and 'practice outcomes'). Endacott *et al.* (2004: 253) call this an 'integrating commentary'. Using the introductions, table of contents and summaries that we suggested in Chapter 3 will help you achieve this level of the hierarchy.

Pause for Thought

• Which is the best way to organize your nursing portfolio?

Shopping trolley

Toast rack

Spinal column

Cake mix

• Why?

Choosing your approach

When considering which of these four approaches is best suited for your portfolio it is clear from the previous section that you should opt for the 'spinal column' or the 'cake mix' approach. However, if you are a novice at portfolio development, these approaches may be too ambitious to begin with, especially if you have a lot of material or many years of experience to cover. In this case we suggest that you avoid the 'shopping trolley' but adopt the 'toast rack' approach which will provide you with a good foundation for development later on as you work towards the 'gold standard' of the 'cake mix'.

Once you have chosen your approach to the management and organization of your portfolio and given attention to the labelling of sections and subsections, you can begin to organize your artefacts and other materials within your chosen structure. The next section is a type of extended case study in which we follow a nurse who is beginning to build a portfolio of his own.

A portfolio in the making

David Omotosa is a general registered nurse employed in a care of the older person unit. David qualified two years ago and is working towards developing his professional nursing portfolio. During his undergraduate programme he created an educational portfolio, however this is his first attempt at a nursing *practice* portfolio. He has chosen to use the NMC domains of competence ('professional values'; 'communication and interpersonal skills'; 'nursing practice and decision-making'; and 'leadership, management and team-working') to structure his portfolio and is starting out with the 'toast rack' approach.

David finds choosing the information to add to his portfolio difficult. He starts by examining his educational and clinical nursing experiences so far, as outlined in his CV. Each element of his education and nursing practice has resulted in learning, and he continues to practise what he has learned since qualifying as a registered nurse. What he actually needs to do now is *unpack the essence of his learning, pull out the key learning experiences* that he would like to discuss and *display the outcome of his learning from his reflections* in his portfolio. In order to do this, David needs to examine the ordinary elements of his nursing practice – things he may have taken for granted as being everyday occurrences. David is advised by his clinical supervisor to start brainstorming his clinical experiences for examples of learning that he might like to focus on in his portfolio. This brainstorming relates directly to the four domains of competence, so that he is focused in his approach.

David decides to focus on the competence of 'professional values' because although he has lots of experience in the other areas this area has particular resonance for him. In order to select specific experiences within this domain for his portfolio, David analyses his learning experiences by asking himself the following questions (Williams 2003):

- *Where did my experience arise?* On the ward? At a conference? From reading?
- *What did I do to enable learning?* Observe? Listen? Take part? Search the literature? Search the web? Make notes?
- *When did I realize I had learned something?* Immediately? When looking over notes? When taking a test?
- *What made this a good learning experience?*

David writes down his answers to these questions in a notebook and makes the observations shown in the panel below.

Where did my experience arise?

Most of my recent learning experience about my personal values took place on P2 ward where I have been working for the last year. We have 30 patients ranging in age from 65 to 98. These patients are being nursed long term in the ward. I haven't attended a specific course in care of the older person, but I did attend a conference recently on dementia. I am sure that I did lots on this topic in college but I can't quite remember what.

What did I do to enable learning?

Other than sitting exams and submitting assignments in college I didn't actively do anything to enable my learning in this specific area of nursing. I can't say I was ever enthused about this field of nursing either. I guess attending the conference on dementia in Cambridge was learning, but I hadn't thought about it that way until now, to be totally honest. I have now been assigned a supervisor on the ward and we talk through care approaches a lot, so I guess I learn there too.

When did I realize I had learned something?

When I initially started working on P2 ward I wasn't really aware of this at first, but I had kind of categorized old people as one large group of infirm people. I bunched them together, thinking that they were all the same, you know, sweet old ladies and grumpy old men, a little hard of hearing. On my ward the charge nurse is very keen that the patients are surrounded as much as possible by their personal effects. I noticed from looking one day at Hilda's photograph that she had once been a most glamorous young lady in the 1920s. I began asking her family about her past and discovered that she had been a very accomplished ballroom dancer, who had won numerous medals and awards. Looking at her now, curled up asleep, it is hard to see this past life. During the day her mind wanders due to her dementia, and there is little talk of her dancing days. At that moment I learned, from experience, not to stereotype people. I feel truly embarrassed now to write this but that was the truth, I didn't see Hilda as a person, I saw her as a patient with dementia. Someone who needed to be washed, fed, toileted and repositioned every now and again. I'm not proud of myself for that. So when I began to think about my patient-centred care and values I realized that I became a nurse because I wanted to give my best to those that needed my help. When I started to think about my present area of practice, I realized that I had let my patients and their families, my colleagues and myself, down. I knew then that I needed to know more about my patients, to find out more about them, their values and where they come from and I needed to treat them respectfully, with consideration for their past and their loved ones. By coincidence, shortly after this experience I attended a training session on 'Respect, dignity and the older person'.

What made this a good learning experience?

What was good about this learning was that it was my own realization. Had it been my supervisor passing a comment to me that I wasn't showing enough respect or taking account of patients' values I might have been quite annoyed about it and perhaps not have believed it, as I thought I was doing a good job until now. Having learned this for myself makes it more believable to me. I have also been triggered to show more empathy now, and this is an inner feeling only I can develop in myself. It was a good coincidence that I attended the training session shortly after my learning experience because I was ready to take in the messages. Hilda and my other patients are more important to me now, and as I get to know them and their families I think my care towards each and every one of them has improved. I have learned a lot about dementia from Hilda's family. I've even seen an improvement in Hilda since we began playing her favourite music in the evenings when she's restless. It's the little things that make a difference.

Honestly I wasn't very enthusiastic about this area of nursing practice initially, but now I really feel that I'm making a difference towards the lives of my patients and their families. My ward manager has even suggested that I undertake a postgraduate diploma in care of the older person and I think I'm really going to enjoy it.

Having unpacked a little of his learning, David entitles the first section in his portfolio 'Professional values'. At this point he doesn't concern himself with the overall introduction to the portfolio or the table of contents. He decides to leave this until he has done a little more work. He then writes out the following extract from the field competencies related to the domain *professional values* from the NMC guidelines and uses this as his introduction.

David Omotosa, RGN BSc

Professional portfolio

Section 1: Professional values

Introduction

'Adult nurses must be able at all times to promote the rights, choices and wishes of all adults and, where appropriate, children and young people, paying particular attention to equality, diversity and the needs of an ageing population. They must be able to work in partnership to address people's needs in all healthcare settings' (NMC 2010: 13).

David decides to focus on the second competence listed within this domain as his first subsection: 'All nurses must practise in a holistic, non-judgemental, caring and sensitive manner that avoids assumptions; supports social inclusion; recognizes and respects individual choice; and acknowledges diversity. Where necessary, they must challenge inequality, discrimination and exclusion from access to care'.

To expand his portfolio David takes some time over the next three weeks to collect the following:

- Module descriptors from his undergraduate programme ('care of the older person'; 'dignity and respect'; 'cultural diversity' and 'communication skills' – total 8 pages).
- An essay on interpersonal caring from his undergraduate nursing programme (5 pages).
- One peer-reviewed paper (5 pages).
- NMC Code of Conduct (2008) (2 pages).
- Local policies (10 pages).
- Personal reflection on a critical incident related to working in a holistic, caring and sensitive manner (1 page).
- Record of conference attendance (1 page).

You will recall from Chapter 1 that the purpose of a portfolio is to 'display achievement of professional competence or learning outcomes and knowledge development' (Timmins 2008: 115). The example that David has written gives us a glimpse of his evidence. However, he needs to analyse and explain his choice of evidence in more detail rather than just including these artefacts in his portfolio. David is conscious that 'individual portfolios are only as good as the evidence they contain' (Cowie 2002: 35) so he works hard to choose evidence that best demonstrates his knowledge and competence in this area.

Using the three phase approach to reflection (see Chapter 2) David begins by critically analysing his knowledge base related to the field competence. He chooses the module descriptors from his undergraduate programme and his essay on interpersonal caring. Using critical reflexivity (Phase 2 of reflection)

David uses the model proposed by Boud *et al.* (1985) (see Chapter 2, p. 36) to re-examine this previous learning, and the result is shown in Table 4.2.

You will see that David was able to draw further elements into his reflection as he went forward, including the peer-reviewed paper and the NMC Code of Conduct.

Table 4.2 Re-examination of David's prior knowledge

Phase of reflection	David's response
1 *Return* to the experience (a brief acknowledgement only, not a full description)	David reads through the module descriptors and his essay and thinks back to his undergraduate programme experience.
2 *Attend* to the feeling (make a note of how you felt)	David is a little shocked at his essay. Although he received a good mark, he had very little experience of nursing at the time, and looking back now it is quite superficial and very theory-based rather than practical. He is also surprised about how much theory was covered that he has actually forgotten.
3 *Associate* (new information resulting from reflection is associated with exisiting knowledge and attitudes)	David re-reads the module descriptors, and takes two books out of the library to read. He updates his current knowledge and tries to consider the practical elements more.
4 *Integrate* (the same new information is integrated with existing knowledge)	David decides that person-centred care, where the older person is treated as a unique individual, with unique needs, is crucial to his current nursing practice. Without this person-centred approach he believes, and now understands, that stereotyping can occur.

5 *Validate* (evidence is used to test any new assumptions resulting from association and integration and ascertain whether there are any inconsistencies or contradictions)	Using new readings and having been to a conference David is sure that his new insight is correct. Healthcare workers in Jones *et al.*'s (2009) study stereotyped older people, and elderly patients received poorer quality care as a result. At the conference, the presenters focused on the importance of caring for patients with dementia, particularly in relation to drawing out the individual needs of the patient, trying to bring back memories from the past and integrating care for the whole family. Reading ward policies and the NMC Code of Conduct confirms to David that this is expected behaviour of every nurse, not just those caring for patients diagnosed with dementia.
6 *Appropriate* (take on the new knowledge as one's own)	Person-centred care that considers the older person as a unique individual is David's priority in this area from now on.

This is only a brief example of the type of discussion that could be included in a portfolio, to demonstrate the way in which material can be drawn together. To further strengthen the content of his portfolio, David decides to reflect on a specific clinical incident (concerning Hilda) using the notes outlined above but placing them within his chosen model of reflection. The result is shown in Table 4.3.

Table 4.3 David's reflection on a critical incident

Phase of reflection	David's notes
1 *Return* to the experience (a brief acknowledgement only, not a full description)	I noticed from looking one day at Hilda's photograph that she had once been a most glamorous young lady in the 1920s. I then discovered, through conversations with her husband and daughter that she had been a very accomplished ballroom dancer, who had won numerous medals and awards. Looking at her now curled up asleep it is hard to see this past life.
2 *Attend* to the feeling (make a note of how you felt)	I feel embarrassment that I hadn't really treated Hilda as an accomplished lady who had lived a full life. I felt sad looking at her now, curled up asleep, having forgotten a lot of her great experiences. I'm also disappointed in myself for not being more caring towards my patients and I wonder if this is because I was not very enthusiastic about working on this unit.
3 *Associate* (new information resulting from reflection is associated with existing knowledge and attitudes)	Having re-read my module descriptors and essay I realize that there is a lot of theoretical information that I can now put into practice. I realize that healthcare staff can lose sight of the person, but must try hard to keep care person-centred.

4 *Integrate* (the same new information is integrated with exisiting knowledge)	Because I feel sad about this and would like to improve the care that I give, I think that taking 15 minutes each day with Hilda, playing old dance music on a CD player, would be helpful. Reminiscence therapy helps people to remember, and this will also help with my person-centred approach. I have made a concerted effort to engage with Hilda and her family and to learn more about her past and what we as nurses can do to individualize the care we give to her and other patients on the unit.
5 *Validate* (evidence is used to test any new assumptions resulting from association and integration and ascertain whether there are any inconsistencies or contradictions)	I have spoken to the charge nurse about my findings from the literature and we have also engaged a music therapist to visit Hilda twice weekly. This therapy seems to be really beneficial for Hilda and other patients on the ward.
6 *Appropriate* (take on the new knowledge as one's own)	Person-centred care for older people has become my approach. I get to know each individual by talking to them and their families. I try to nurse the whole person, considering how they were in their life prior to admission, and try to be respectful at all times. I now understand the importance of demonstrating person-centred respectful care in all my actions.

Observation as evidence

To build up additional evidence, David arranged for his supervisor to observe a morning of his practice and comment on it. He also wrote up an account of this for the relevant section of his portfolio, and asked his supervisor to co-sign it. An outline of the format David used is shown in Figure 4.5. The evidence from David's supervisor will serve to validate his own assumptions in his reflections, i.e. that his approach is person-centred.

	Comment
Date	
The learning experience(s)	
Morning nursing care of 10 older clients in long-term care	
Demonstration of Practice in a holistic, non-judgemental, caring and sensitive manner that avoids assumptions, supports social inclusion, recognizes and respects individual choice and acknowledges diversity. Where necessary, challenge inequality, discrimination and exclusion from access to care.	
Signature:	
Observer's signature:	

Figure 4.5 Sample evidence form for direct observation.

Once this phase of reflection is complete, David moves on to Phase 3 (critical action). He decides that he will continue to have ongoing supervision at work in relation to this particular domain, and that he will attend a short course to improve his knowledge and understanding in this area.

Using his portfolio as a vehicle for professional development, David now reconsiders his work-based learning in terms of:

- his knowledge of practice (including relevant policy and legislation);
- his reflexive account;
- what action he took/needs to take.

He brings all the items related to these elements together, including his reflections, and then creates a summary of the whole subsection.

In this example of David we outlined some of the types of evidence that can be included within a subsection of a portfolio. There are many other types, and some of these are outlined in the box below.

Suggested evidence for inclusion in a portfolio

- An outline and discussion of focused reading that you have completed. This includes a brief list of references related to a topic, which are read, and brief notes made on each.

- Description of practice project. This includes a summary of key points on a practice-related project.

- Description of clinical experiences and reflections on these.

- Description of observations from practice.

- Testimonies (client or other staff).

- Certificates of attendance at educational events.

(continued overleaf)

- Evidence of involvement in committee work related to your role and/or reflection on this.

- Evidence of membership of professional organizations.

- 'Thank you' cards.

- Competence documentation.

- Attendance records.

- Summary of guidelines and protocols, or some aspect of these.

- Summary of patient information leaflets.

- Summary of research article related to practice.

- Summary of prior classroom learning/module descriptor/curriculum content on a topic.

- Photographs, videos or DVD (with permission) of skills performed.

- Notes on peer-reviewed observed practice.

- Reflections.

- Case studies.

Documenting practice as evidence

If you are preparing documentation so that your supervisor can observe you in practice, other than when you are involved in a structured course of study, it should be brief. The staff member concerned should not be placed in a position where they are in any way held accountable for your competence or practice. The documentation is simply a record stating that you were observed and that in the observer's opinion you were safe and professional in that practice. Documenting your practice in this way, done correctly, is a very useful tool when you wish to demonstrate the areas in which you are accomplished and those on which you need to improve.

Another way of documenting your practice as evidence is the testimonial. Here you ask a colleague if they are willing to compose a short (about 250 words) testimonial about a specific area of your practice. You may be pleasantly surprised about how glowing such a report actually is. We are all inclined to underemphasize our achievements at times, or to focus on our weakness. While there is certainly merit in building up areas where weaknesses exist, we also need to acknowledge our strengths. This in turn will help us in acknowledging that we also have work to do on our weaker points.

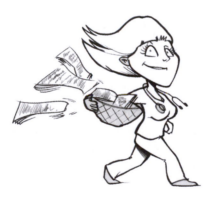

Making sense of your portfolio

Making sense of your portfolio is ultimately about being creative and making it your own. But it is also about how the over-arching narrative will explain why you chose to include certain artefacts and not others, and how each section and subsection is elaborated by your commentary as it arises. Unlike an essay, the portfolio commentary, in which you 'talk' to your reader, does not need to be particularly formal. At the minimum it may only consist of a few lines at the beginning and end of each section. The best advice here is to say it how it is, but say it clearly and concisely. An example of an opening commentary from a portfolio section concerned with ethical issues is given in the panel below, to give you a flavour.

> When I moved to Burnett Ward, I was really surprised by the many uncomfortable situations I found myself in. I hadn't really seen a real-life ethical dilemma, as my previous experience was in outpatients. What I learned in my training all seemed a bit theoretical to me at the time, and now I feel a real need to brush up on this learning. This is why I chose to look at my knowledge of contemporary ethical issues in this section of my portfolio. A lot of what I'm looking at relates to me reassessing what I learned as a student and trying to apply this to my current practice. I have also included some reflections on my practice and some summaries on reading that I have recently completed.

In addition to, or as an alternative to, the commentary, you may choose to include visual aids such as diagrams or mind-maps. Remember there are no strict rules about the format of your portfolio, so feel free to be creative. For example, if you are working with clients with intellectual disabilities and you have been involved with their craft work, you may like to include examples of this, or photographs of it to support your commentary.

Conclusion

By now you should have developed a good idea of how you want to structure your portfolio and the approach you will take. If you are new to portfolios, we recommend starting with the 'toast rack' and developing from there to the 'spinal column' and finally to the 'cake mix' formula. This chapter has provided information on all the approaches along with an example of a portfolio being developed (by David) and advice on documenting your practice and making sense of your portfolio via your ongoing commentary for the benefit of your reader (and yourself when you look back over your work in the future).

The next chapter focuses on the practical and ethical issues of what, and what not, to include in your portfolio.

Summary

- Be organized.
- Allocate specific time for your portfolio development and stick to it.
- Pick particular themes or domains on which to focus.
- Start by aiming for the toast rack approach.
- Remember to analyse your evidence and present it in a logical manner.
- Introduce and summarize your sections and subsections via your commentary.
- Aim for the 'spinal column' approach but work towards the 'cake mix' in the long run.

References

Boud, D. *et al.* (1985) Promoting reflection in learning: a model, in D. Boud, D. Walker and R. Keogh, *Reflection: Turning Experience into Learning*. London: Kogan Page.

Cowie, A. (2002) Portfolio development for nurses and healthcare assistants, *Nursing Management*, 8(10): 34–5.

Endacott, R., Gray, M.A., Jasper, M., McMullan, M., Miller, C., Scholes, J. and Webb, C. (2004) Using portfolios in the assessment of learning and competence: the impact of four models, *Nurse Education in Practice* 4(4): 250–7.

Jones, S.M., Vahia, I.V., Cohen, C.I., Hindi, A. and Nurhussein, M. (2009) A pilot study to assess attitudes, behaviors, and inter-office communication by psychiatrists and primary care providers in the care of older adults with schizophrenia, *International Journal of Geriatric Psychiatry*, 24(3): 254–60.

NMC (Nursing and Midwifery Council) (2008) *The Code: Standards of Conduct, Performance and Ethics for Nurses and Midwives*. London: NMC.

NMC (Nursing and Midwifery Council) (2010) *Standards for Pre-registration Nursing Education*. London: NMC.

Timmins, F. (2008) *Making Sense of Portfolios: An Introduction to Portfolio Use for Nursing Students*. Maidenhead: Open University Press.

Williams, M. (2003) Developing portfolios for peri-operative nurses, *Nursing Standard*, 18(1): 46–55.

5 Ethical and professional issues

By the end of this chapter you will:

○ Be able to review the content of your portfolio in the light of what has been discussed so far.
○ Be aware of ethical issues that you may encounter when developing your portfolio.
○ Be aware of professional and legal considerations.
○ Understand some possible solutions to some of the challenges faced in these areas.

This chapter addresses a common challenge of portfolio development for nurses in relation to what to actually keep in the portfolio and the practical and ethical issues associated with your choices. It addresses the decision-making required in this process and offers practical advice.

Reviewing the content

We have provided some suggestions about how to order and categorize the contents of your portfolio in Chapters 3 and 4. In essence, your portfolio is an ongoing record of all you have achieved as a consequence of critical reflection on your nursing practice.

Portfolios are a self-directive method of evaluating your achievement of clinical competence through the use of critical reflection. By this stage you will have accumulated a considerable number of artefacts which may include:

- Year exam/assignment results from your certificate/degree/diploma
- Individual essays and assignments
- Projects
- Mandatory training (e.g. in cardiopulmonary resuscitation – CPR)
- Skills training
- Prizes and awards
- Final certificate/diploma/degree
- Study day/conference attendance
- Results of online/distance learning modules

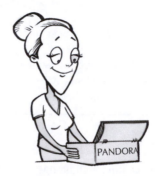

So which of these items should remain in your portfolio? If you were to include them all it is likely that the logical structure you have imposed as a result of reading Chapters 3 and 4 would be difficult to maintain. To begin with, bear in mind that all your award achievements (certificates/diplomas/ degrees) can be listed in your CV, which should always be included. However, specific awards and evidence of achievement may be included if you answer 'yes' to the following questions:

- Have I identified an organized structure for my portfolio? *If the answer is 'no', you need to read back over Chapters 3 and 4 and decide on an organizing framework before you consider the place for your achievements. If the answer is 'yes', proceed to the next question.*
- Does this piece of evidence fit within the framework I have chosen for my portfolio? *Apply this to each piece of evidence you have. If the answer is*

'no' then the evidence concerned belongs in your 'holding area' (i.e. your box file or computer file for this purpose). If the answer is 'yes', retain the evidence for consideration within your final portfolio.

Once you have organized and categorized your achievements according to your framework, you can file them temporarily within each section until you have dedicated time to examine the evidence in more detail. This will involve considering whether or not the evidence has a logical place in your portfolio. Although the evidence might reasonably fit, remember that your portfolio has to make sense. It is also important that it does not grow too big; otherwise it becomes unmanageable for you and unwieldy for others to read. At this point you will need to have outlined the sections and subsections that you will use. Consider whether the evidence:

- is relevant to the chosen section;
- is linked specifically to the competence;
- demonstrates your proficiency/achievement in the competence.

If the evidence fits with all the above considerations, then it is suitable for inclusion at this point in your portfolio. Remember however that the portfolio is a journey and not a precise science and therefore at some point later on you may change your mind about the evidence you decide to include, depending on how the portfolio is coming together. A crucial point is whether or not you have too much evidence related to a specific competence. If this is the case you will be well advised to consider what is the *best* evidence. Ask yourself which evidence of achievement *best* demonstrates your proficiency in the chosen competence.

Writing in your portfolio

Writing, as you will have realized by now, is a significant element in your portfolio. In Chapter 2 we introduced the concept of writing out your reflections on practice and including these in your portfolio. In Chapter 4 we emphasized the importance of including a dialogue or commentary within your portfolio – a continuous 'conversation' throughout that helps to link the sections together. Other writing will include, for example, ward profiles, nursing experiences and case studies. However, all these types of writing can be placed into two distinct categories:

- reflective writing;

  and

- analytical writing.

Naturally, reflective writing emerges when you begin to apply your chosen model of reflection. Analytical writing takes place when you are drawing your portfolio together, or critically analysing your experiences and achievements.

There are certain guidelines that need to be followed when you engage in reflective and analytical writing in your portfolio. Your writing should:

- be a truthful and honest account;
- be your own work, not copied from other sources without correct citation;
- be from your own perspective;
- not cause harm to others;
- not be used as a substitute for the usual communication channels or reporting mechanisms applied in practice.

In addition to achievements and awards, a great deal of time is spent writing about clinical practice as part of the portfolio. There are also important ethical considerations that need to be taken into account when considering clinical practice as evidence.

Ethical considerations

Caring is the essence of nursing practice, so your portfolio will relate to your experience of caring for patients in the real world. However, nursing as a profession is bound by ethical and legal codes that guide all practice. Thus, you need to consider the ethical and legal implications of the following:

- including policies/procedures/standards/guidelines from your health employer;
- reflecting on incidents in practice;

- writing up case studies;
- discussing ways of working (e.g. team meetings, performance appraisal)

You will also need to ensure that your writing within the portfolio is subject to the same job description guidelines, ethical and legal codes that guide your nursing practice (Jasper 2006).

Ethical dilemmas

Although the NMC Code of Conduct stipulates the need to respect patient choice, there are occasions when you may not agree with the patient's decision and this is when ethical conflict of interest or ethical dilemmas can arise. This is something that you may wish to write about in your portfolio. Acting as an ethical practitioner can be very difficult, and you may find it useful to discuss difficult ethical situations with your reflective friend, asking questions such as:

- Did I really understand and respect my patient's position in this dilemma?
- What factors impacted on my approach?
- Was there anything I could have done differently to help my patient make a more informed decision about the treatment or care?
- How do I now feel about the patient's decision, or mine?

In the following scenario, Claire has written out her concerns about one of the patients in her care.

Scenario: Claire and Susan

Susan is a 44-year-old mother of three children aged, 4, 6 and 10. I was allocated to her care. Susan is the same age as me and we are both mothers of young children. We actually got on very well. Susan was admitted for investigations for bone pain, anaemia and weakness. She told me she just felt that all she needed was a holiday in the sun, but when she collapsed her husband insisted she make an appointment to see her GP, and her GP then referred her to the local hospital. So here she was, admitted for investigations. She laughed and said that she was finally getting her well-earned break.

And then the devastating news came - Susan was diagnosed with multiple myeloma (MM). She asked if I could explain what I knew about this type of cancer. I informed her I would get as much information as I could. That afternoon when I finished my shift I went to the hospital library and asked the librarian to help me find articles on MM. As soon as I started to read the literature I knew Susan was in 'trouble'. Rice and Sheridan (2000) explained that the disease is fatal and intervention is directed at symptom control. I knew the doctors had given Susan some information about her treatment options but I also felt that Susan was hoping I would be able to give her more positive feedback.

I was in a dilemma: I did not want to tell Susan how fatal her prognosis was. I didn't sleep the night before I was next on duty. I brought the Rice and Sheridan article with me because I knew Susan had the right to know about her condition and read about it for herself. I had also accessed some websites with patient stories so that Susan could see how other people with the condition were managing. I gave Susan the literature and her husband brought in her laptop. I asked Susan if she wanted me to stay with her and explain the information, but she said she'd prefer to read the literature and look at the websites with her husband. She thanked me and because I respected her right to privacy I left her and her husband alone to read. When I returned to her later in the morning to help her wash, she asked me to leave the room.

I have been qualified for four years and have never had such a terrible experience. I did as she asked and later that afternoon the consultant informed us that Susan had decided she did not want treatment and was discharging herself from the hospital. I was devastated and blamed myself. I couldn't believe that Susan would give up on her life, her children and her family so easily. I would fight tooth and nail to live for my children. I just couldn't understand why a mother would give up so easily.

Claire's situation would be difficult for any nurse to deal with. Claire decided to use this incident as a learning event for a portfolio entry. She began by choosing an appropriate domain of competence, in this case, 'professional values'. Claire reflected that she had a duty of care to Susan, which she fulfilled, because she tried to act in her patient's best interests by providing her with the relevant information to make an informed decision about her treatment options. Susan decided not to undergo treatment, which Claire felt was the wrong decision. She examined the reasons for these feelings – perhaps they were related to her own personal identification with Susan as a mother? Claire reflected that she had attempted to build a trusting relationship with Susan and had acted as an advocate by identifying literature and websites that Susan could read and understand. She had also asked Susan if she wanted her to explain the literature to her, and then gave her and her husband the privacy they requested. Despite all this, Claire was left feeling very upset at her patient's reaction. Claire set out her reflection in a way that will now be familiar to you, and this is shown in Table 5.1.

Table 5.1 Claire's reflection

Phase of reflection	Claire's response
1 *Return* to the experience (a brief acknowledgement only, not a full description)	Susan was a 44-year-old mother of three in my care diagnosed with MM. I knew the doctors had given her some information about her treatment options, but I felt that she was hoping I would be able to give her more positive information. I was in a dilemma – I did not want to tell Susan how fatal her prognosis was, but I wanted to be able to inform her appropriately. Susan later discharged herself and refused treatment.
2 *Attend* to the feeling (make a note of how you felt)	I felt really sad at first when I heard of Susan's diagnosis. Being a mother of young children the same age as Susan's, I kept imagining what it must be like. I cried and couldn't sleep for thinking about it.
3 *Associate* (new information resulting from reflection is associated with existing knowledge and attitudes)	Having read back over my notes on communication, ethical dilemmas and the Code of Conduct, I see that it is a patient's choice to make an informed decision regarding their care or treatment. My feelings about it were related to my overt identification with Susan as a person, and what decision I

	might make in that situation. I learned that nurses ought to be more detached in professional therapeutic relationships and that patient choice is paramount. I also read back through information that I have on beliefs about health and how these are very individual and can affect individuals' approach to health behaviours. Thus my health beliefs are not the same as others.
4 *Integrate* (the same new information is integrated with existing knowledge)	Because I feel sad about this situation, I know that I need to use these feelings to develop appropriate empathy and sympathy for patients rather than becoming upset when patients make their own choice.
5 *Validate* (evidence is used to test any new assumptions resulting from association and integration and ascertain whether there are any inconsistencies or contradictions)	In my ongoing practice, I notice that a professional therapeutic relationship is better than an overly professional one. I also notice that my initial reading was restricted to the patient's condition only, and not the wider issues of relationships, empowerment, understanding and choice. From speaking later with the consultant I found out that Susan was ultimately well informed about her condition, and was very happy with her decision.

(continued overleaf)

Table 5.1 Continued

Phase of reflection	Claire's response
6 *Appropriate* (take on the new knowledge as one's own)	*In relation to the standards of practice required of me as a nurse I need to consider:* *1 Communication and interpersonal skills* *2 Personal values in more detail for my portfolio.*

Even though Claire was very emotional about this experience, her reflection, while not discounting this, focuses on new learning about herself and her nursing practice. At the end of the reflection Claire is just about ready for the next phase of reflection – critical action, and you will be asked to give some consideration to the type of critical action that Claire might take in the next pause for thought.

You may have noticed that Claire's experience crosses *two* domains of competence, 'professional values' and 'communication and interpersonal skills'. As a result she could consider utilizing this reflection, and the subsequent learning, across two sections of her portfolio. The same could easily happen to you: you begin by reflecting on one aspect of practice, only to reveal another in the process. In this way your portfolio can sometimes 'build itself'.

Prioritizing care

Prioritizing care is another ethical dilemma you may face in today's healthcare environment. With moratoriums on nursing recruitment, bed closures, financial and budgetary constraints it can be difficult to provide the effective and most satisfactory patient care that you would give in an ideal world. These factors need to be taken into account when analysing reflections on practice, particularly in relation to your maintenance or attainment of clinical competence. The culture of your healthcare organization will also have a significant impact on the care you provide. A useful model is provided by

Pause for Thought

- What would you have done if you had been in Claire's position?

- How would you help Claire through this reflection if she asked you to be her reflective friend?

- In what way could this situation impact on Claire's future nursing practice?

- What critical action do you think Claire should take?

- Have you ever had an experience where your views on care delivery/health promotion differed from the expressed needs of the patient? Write down you experience. Use the results from this pause for thought as a portfolio entry.

Johnson and Scholes (1999) and is known as the *cultural web model* (see Figure 5.1).

The model provides an alternative way for you to reflect on organizational issues. Begin by looking at each element of the 'cultural web' separately. Ask

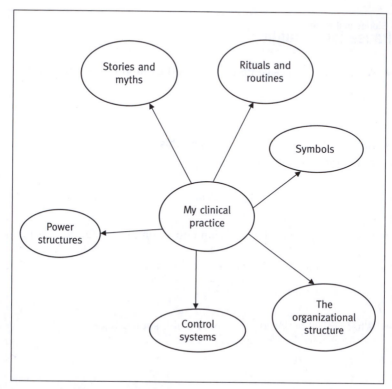

Figure 5.1 The cultural web model.

yourself key questions such as those shown in Figure 5.2 to help you establish what you believe to be important within each element in your organization.

Once you have considered these questions, with your reflective friend if you like, you can begin to make more sense of the impact of issues such as power structures, myths and stories and, in particular 'routines and rituals' on the care you give to your patients. You should attempt to identify how these factors can impact on your ethical decision-making process. Read the scenario on page 114 and consider the ethical decision-making process involved.

Stories and myths

- What is the reputation of your workplace, ward or hospital?
- What stories do people currently tell about your organization?
- What do these stories say about your workplace philosophy or beliefs?
- What stories do your colleagues tell new people who join?
- Who are the heroes, villains and mavericks in these stories?
- How do these factors impact on the care you give to your patients?

Rituals and routines

- What do patients expect when they enter your workplace?
- What do your colleagues expect?
- What would be immediately obvious if it was changed?
- What behaviour do routines encourage?
- When a new problem is encountered, what rules do people apply when they solve it?
- What core beliefs do these rituals reflect?
- How do these factors impact on the care you give to your patients?

Symbols

- Is nursing-specific jargon or language used?
- Are there any status symbols on your ward/in your hospital?
- What image is associated with your workplace, looking at this specifically from the separate viewpoints of clients and staff?
- How do these factors impact on the care you give to your patients?

(continued overleaf)

Organizational structure

- Is the structure of your workplace flat or hierarchical? Formal or informal?

- Where are the formal lines of authority?

- Are there informal lines?

- How do these factors impact on the care you give to your patients?

Control systems

- What process or procedure has the strongest controls? Weakest controls?

- Is your workplace generally loosely or tightly controlled?

- Do employees get rewarded for good work or penalized for poor work?

- What reports are issued to keep control of operations, finance, etc.?

- How do these factors impact on the care you give to your patients?

Power structures

- Who has the real power in your workplace?

- What do these people believe and champion within your workplace?

- Who makes or influences decisions?

- How is this power used or abused?

- How do these factors impact on the care you give to your patients?

Figure 5.2 Questions to consider.

Scenario: Ward routines

In a care of the older person ward the unit manager insists on having all patients washed and sitting out by 10 a.m. This is ward routine and not evidenced-based practice. As a consequence you may be faced with an ethical dilemma regarding prioritizing your care: if you spend valuable time speaking to a patient you may not achieve the goal of having all your patients washed and sitting out by 10 a.m.

You don't want your nurse manager to think you are attempting to avoid work by sitting 'chatting' to a patient when your nursing colleagues are working hard washing patients and getting them out of bed. If you do stop to chat to a patient you may then need the assistance of a colleague to help you finish the ward routine and they may feel put out as a result.

- In these or similar circumstances you have to weigh up the benefits and risks of prioritizing your nursing care.
- You need to be able to justify your actions to your unit manager and/or nursing colleagues.
- With the help of your reflective friend you may be able to propose a change to the ward routine and rituals.
- Your reflective portfolio can help you identify such issues. Sharing your thoughts with your reflective friend or your colleagues may well result in positive changes to your nursing practice.

To conclude this section, we offer you a list of broad guidelines in relation to the ethical issues surrounding portfolio entries and writing. Educators sometimes express concern at the potential for students to 'overstep the mark' (albeit unwittingly) in this respect (e.g. Burns and Bulman 2000). There have even been calls for a code of ethics to apply to any writing or documentation about patients outside the clinical area (Hargreaves 1997). However, this type of specific guidance is notably absent from portfolio guidelines emerging from within the profession (e.g. NCNM 2009). The best advice we can give is to manage your portfolio as an extension of your professional practice, and be aware of all professional, legal and ethical requirements that guide our nursing practice:

- Always ensure you have patient consent to use information in relation to them.
- Always maintain confidentiality and anonymity.
- Always keep your portfolio safe and secure.
- Always obtain permission to use local documents.
- Make full use of the NMC Code of Conduct.

The NMC Code of Conduct

The NMC (2008) Code of Conduct provides invaluable guidance when it comes to matters of ethics and professionalism in nursing practice: just the things that you need to apply to your portfolio as well as your day-to-day practice. As you may already be aware, the Code requires that you:

- make the care of people your first concern, treating them as individuals and respecting their dignity;
- work with others to protect and promote the health and well-being of those in your care, their families and carers, and the wider community;
- provide a high standard of practice and care at all times;
- be open and honest, act with integrity and uphold the reputation of your profession.

There must be evidence of these standards of care within your portfolio. Specific points for consideration for portfolio entries relating to patients are:

- *Patient choice:* did the patient consent to their care being included in my portfolio?
- *Non-discriminatory approach:* are my comments appropriate in this regard?
- *Critical reflection:* did I provide a high standard of care at all times? If not, have I addressed this through critical action?

In relation to the last point, it is important to remember that it is usually your own nursing practice that you are writing about in your portfolio, although brief references are sometimes made to other staff. Incidents of your own poor practice, if these are identified in your portfolio, need to be managed by critical action. You may need to report such occurrences to your manager, following local/national procedures in relation to this. Remember, any professional nurse reading your portfolio (such as those in the NMC, or your reflective friend) is under the same obligation to follow through on incidents of poor, unsafe, unethical or illegal practice as you are.

> **Remember!**
>
> Incidents of your own poor practice identified in your portfolio need to be managed by critical action.

Upholding *high standards of practice* is crucial in your role as a nurse. Any deviation from this should be, and is likely to be, dealt with within the clinical arena, at the time of, or close to the time of, the occurrence. In reality it is unusual, although not impossible, for these events to come to light in your portfolio. However, it is important to keep the NMC Code uppermost in your mind at all times when working on your portfolio, so that you are not tempted to utilize it as a 'secondary reporting device' for episodes of poor standards of practice.

> **Remember!**
>
> Your portfolio is not a personal record or diary in which you can unburden yourself about incidents of poor practice.

Professional and legal considerations

As a professional nurse, you are personally accountable for actions and omissions in your practice and must always be able to justify your decisions.

However, despite our best efforts, errors and mistakes will and do occur. It is important to reflect on medical errors and learn from your mistakes. In general such situations are dealt with between the staff member and the organization and should not be used for portfolio purposes. To do so may cause harm to you, the patient concerned or your organization, depending on the nature and context of the situation.

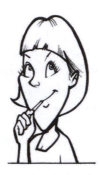

Errors often occur due to a lack of knowledge, workload issues, staffing levels, emotional and physical factors, not knowing or not adhering to policies and procedures, shift work and distractions or disruptions during a shift (Esi Owusu Agyemang and While 2010). It is very important that such situations are acknowledged, recorded, investigated and improvements made to facilitate better and more professional care. Let us consider a scenario that highlights the legal issues that may be inherent in a portfolio entry.

Scenario: Antonia

I have been qualified for 15 years and work part-time in the outpatient department. One morning I came on duty and Nursing Administration phoned to inform us that one staff nurse was to go to the A&E department. I was chosen. I argued with my colleagues that I was not happy to work in the A&E

department and we agreed to draw straws over who should go. I couldn't believe it when I drew the short straw. To be honest I was not at all pleased, but I didn't feel I could argue any further as my colleagues had been fair in the selection process.

When I arrived at the A&E department, there was chaos all around me. There were patients on trolleys in the corridor, people sleeping in the waiting room. I didn't know what to do or where to begin. The charge nurse greeted me by simply stating, 'At last - we expected you 30 minutes ago! You're looking after the five patients in bays one to five, and you can get a handover from the nurse who is currently looking after them.' I didn't get a second to tell her I'd never worked in A&E before and I was very anxious.

The nurse gave me a very brief handover, and left me to it! I also didn't know any of the nurses working in the department so felt very alone and unsure of myself. This was an unusual feeling for me, having significant nursing experience, albeit in a different environment. I told myself to just get on with it!

The patients needed their morning medication, so I located their drug kardex and proceeded to give them their medication. I mixed up the patients' medications and administered two patients the wrong drugs. It wasn't until one of the patients asked me what the 'new' tablets were that I realized my mistake. I had given cardiac drugs and potassium to the wrong patient and the other patient received a narcotic that wasn't prescribed for them.

I almost collapsed when I realized my error and immediately alerted the charge nurse. She was absolutely furious and then I began to cry. We quickly notified the patients' medical teams and the patients were monitored very carefully as a consequence. One of the patients was transferred to the resuscitation section to be carefully monitored by telemetry. I had to inform the patients and their families about the errors, inform Nursing Administration and complete two very detailed incident forms. I was then told to take the remainder of the shift off and to report to the Director of Nursing office before duty the following morning. Before I left the emergency department I overheard the charge nurse saying, 'If this is what happens when Nursing Administration give us relief we'd be better off coping on our own.' I went straight out to my car and burst into tears.

Antonia later phoned a colleague and discussed the incident with her. Her colleague advised her to write down her thoughts about the incident and they met to discuss the situation. Her colleague asked her some critical questions to enable Antonia to analyse the situation in an objective manner. Antonia used Rolfe *et al.*'s (2001) model ('What?'; 'So what?'; 'Now what?') (see Cronin and Rawlings-Anderson 2004: 158) to analyse the day's events. This is a good model for spur of the moment reflection on action, and using the three headings Antonia asked herself the following.

What happened?

- What was the problem?
- What was my role in the situation?
- What was I trying to achieve?
- What action did I take?
- What was the response of others?
- What were the consequences for the patients/for me/for others?

- What feelings were evoked for all involved?
- What was good and bad about the experience?

So what?

- What did the situation tell me about my patient care and personal attitude?
- What was I thinking about when I acted in the situation?
- What did I base my actions on?
- What knowledge did I bring to the situation – experiential, personal and scientific?
- What could I or should I have done to make the situation better?
- What new understanding emerged following the situation?
- What were the broader issues inherent in the situation?

What now?

- What can I do to improve my patient care, make things better, resolve the situation and feel better in myself?
- What broader issues need to be considered if my actions are to be successful?
- What might the consequences of further action entail?

The important thing to draw from Antionia's reflection is that she did not use the resulting material in her portfolio because she was potentially guilty of non-compliance with the NMC Code. Despite this, through her reflection Antonia learned critical lessons from this experience in terms of being a more assertive communicator, working under stressful circumstances and the reality of human error in clinical practice.

Conclusion

This chapter should have made you more aware of some of the ethical and legal issues that may arise as a consequence of reflecting on your nursing practice via a portfolio.

In the next chapter we look at ways you can further refine the content of your portfolio as it develops.

Summary

- What you include or remove from your portfolio is a matter of personal choice.
- Your writing within the portfolio will either be *reflective* or *analytical*.
- Ethical and legal dilemmas are part of nursing practice. Observation of codes of conduct and any other procedural and legal guidelines is essential when considering what to include in your portfolio.
- The portfolio is not a substitute for formal or informal reporting mechanisms. The nurse has a duty of care that must be discharged in the clinical setting.

References

Burns, S. and Bulman, C. (2000) *Reflective Practice in Nursing: The Growth of Professional Practitioner*, 2nd edn. London: Blackwell Science.

Cronin, P. and Rawlings-Anderson, K. (2004) *Knowledge for Contemporary Nursing Practice*. London: Mosby.

Esi Owusu Agyemang R. and While A. (2010) Medication errors: types, causes and impact on nursing practice, *British Journal of Nursing*, 19(6): 380–5.

Hargreaves, J. (1997) Using patients: exploring the ethical dimension of reflective practice in education, *Journal of Advanced Nursing*, 25(2): 223–8.

Jasper, M. (2006) Portfolios and the use of evidence, in M. Jasper (ed.) *Professional Development, Reflection and Decision-making*. Oxford: Blackwell.

Johnson, G. and Scholes, K. (1999) *Exploring Corporate Strategy*, 5th edn. Harlow: Prentice Hall.

NCNM (The National Council for the Professional Development of Nursing and Midwifery) (2009) *Guidelines for Portfolio Development for Nurses and Midwives*, www.ncnm.ie/default.asp?V_DOC_ID=2431&V_LANG_ID=5 (accessed 19 October 2010).

NMC (Nursing and Midwifery Council) (2008) *The Code: Standards of Conduct, Performance and Ethics for Nurses and Midwives*. London: NMC.

Rice, D. and Sheridan, C.A. (2000) Nursing care of patients with multiple myeloma: a paradigm for the needs of special populations, *Clinical Journal of Oncology Nursing*, 5(3): 89–93.

Rolfe, G., Freshwater, D. and Jasper, M. (2001) *Critical Reflection in Nursing and the Helping Professions: A User's Guide*. Basingstoke: Palgrave Macmillan.

Refining your portfolio

6

By the end of this chapter you will:

○ Have further refined your portfolio's sections and subsections.
○ Have a greater understanding of the use of competency frameworks and the meaning of 'competence'.
○ Have read through an example from a nursing student's portfolio.
○ Have learned some techniques for writing up your portfolio.
○ Be better prepared to overcome the inevitable challenges you will face.

It is now time to further refine your portfolio. We return to some areas we have already discussed and look at them in more detail with the aim of helping you to move on the the next stage of portfolio development.

Sections and subsections

You should by now be aware that in order to organize your portfolio you need to think about a specific framework. For example, you could divide your port-folio into three sections: personal details and/or your CV; a summary of your nursing experience; and a focus on selected domains of competence or other themes of your choice.

Depending on your choice of an over-arching framework (e.g. domains of competence), and the depth at which you decide to explore these, you will create at least three other relevant sections. These may be further divided into subsections, depending on your choice of framework. Your over-arching framework should now begin to look like Table 6.1.

Table 6.1 Over-arching framework for a portfolio

Section 1	CV	
Section 2	Nursing experience	
Section 3	Domain of competence 1	*Subsection A* *Subsection B* *Subsection C*
Section 4	Domain of competence 2	*Subsection A* *Subsection B* *Subsection C*
Section 5	Domain of competence 3	*Subsection A* *Subsection B* *Subsection C*

We will now expand on our rationale for applying this framework to your nursing portfolio, and the potential use of competencies as an organizing 'superstructure'.

Competency frameworks and the meaning of 'competence'

'Competence' is increasingly used in undergraduate nurse education pro-grammes to describe the knowledge, skills and behaviour required of a practising nurse upon registration. Achievement of required competencies by nursing students forms the backbone of both student assessment and ulti-mately nurse registration in the UK. On this basis, competencies drive and structure undergraduate nursing curricula to a considerable extent. Compe-tence frameworks are increasingly also used to structure post-registration knowledge and skill development, as well as role expansion. Therefore, it makes sense to structure your learning, and your description of it, around these 'key pillars' of the nursing profession.

Clinical competence and competency

The issue of developing clinical competence is a key theme in policy documents from the statutory bodies guiding nursing practice worldwide (Storey 2001). Definitions of competence from national and international nursing bodies and the literature include the following:

> Competence is the ability of the registered nurse or midwife to practise safely and effectively, fulfilling his/her professional responsibility within his/her scope of practice.
>
> (An Bord Altranais 2000: 7)

> the skills and ability to practise safely and effectively without the need of direct supervision.
>
> (UKCC 1999: 35)

> Competence requires knowledge, appropriate attitudes and observable mechanical or intellectual skills which, together, account for the ability to deliver a specified professional service.
>
> (WHO 1988: 68)

Is there a difference between competence and *competencies*? Certainly there is sometimes confusion between the two terms. Zhang *et al.* (2001) make a neat distinction by saying that *competencies* are the knowledge, skills, motives and attitudes required in order to achieve *competence*. Such knowledge and skills include trust, knowledge of one's own limitations, caring, communication skills, adaptability, critical thinking, building on knowledge and skills, and demonstrating effecting action (Girot 1993; Valloze 2009). Figure 6.1 provides an outline of some contemporary nurse competencies, some of which you will already have come across in our discussions in Chapter 3.

As you can see from Figure 6.1, there are many competencies that you can focus on in your portfolio, although as we have said you should focus on a framework for competence that resonates with you and that you feel defines your nursing practice.

Generic competencies for nurses (NMC 2010)

- Professional values
- Communication and interpersonal skills
- Nursing practice and decision-making
- Leadership, management and team working

Generic competencies for nurses (An Bord Altranais 2004)

- Professional/ethical practice
- Holistic approaches to care and the integration of knowledge
- Interpersonal relationships
- Organization and management of care
- Personal and professional development

Clinical nursing specialist competencies (NCNM 2008a)

- Clinical focus
- Patient/client advocate
- Education and training
- Audit and research
- Consultant

Advanced nurse specialist competencies (NCNM 2008b)

- Autonomy in clinical practice
- Expert practice
- Professional and clinical leadership
- Research

Competencies for nurse managers (Rush *et al.* 2000)

- Building and managing relationships
- Communication and influencing skills

(continued overleaf)

- Practitioner competence and professional credibility

- Promoting evidence-based decision-making

- Service initiation and innovation

- Resilience and composure

- Sustained personal commitment

- Integrity and ethical stance

Front-level manager

- Planning and organization of activities and resources

- Building and leading the team

- Leading on clinical practice and service quality

Middle-level manager

- Proactive approach to planning

- Effective coordination of resources

- Empowering/enabling leadership

- Setting and monitoring performance standards

- Negotiation skills

Top-level manager

- Strategic and system thinking

- Establishing policy, systems and structures

- Leading on vision and values

- Stepping up to the corporate agenda

- Development approach to staff

Figure 6.1 A range of nurse competency frameworks in current use.

Pause for Thought

- If you are a nurse manager it would probably be better to focus on the development or maintenance of the competencies outlined by Rush *et al*. If you are employed as a clinical nurse specialist you will probably focus on one of the competencies defined by the NCNM.

A nursing student's portfolio

Pause for Thought

Write down your concerns relating to developing your reflective nursing portfolio. Consider the following questions and if need be refer back to previous chapters to find the answers.

- How can I demonstrate that I am a competent nurse?

- How will I choose an incident for reflection that is appropriate?

- How do I actually write about the incident in my portfolio?

- How will I deal with ethical or legal issues that arise?

- Who will read my portfolio?

- Does it all need to be true?

To move the process on, we now look at Stephanie's attempt at reflection as a final year nursing student using the model proposed by Gibbs (1988) (see Chapter 2). Her notes on a specific incident are given in Table 6.2.

Stephanie found this model useful in identifying her learning and dealing with her emergent feelings about the event. When considering how this reflection might fit within the portfolio, Stephanie decided that the following themes had emerged:

- Providing holistic nursing care
- Decision-making
- Being part of an effective team
- Developing and maintaining effective communication
- Developing self-confidence

Table 6.2 Stephanie's reflection

1 Describe the event	I was recently looking after a terminally ill patient called Anne (pseudonym) who suddenly and severely became short of breath while I was walking her back from the bathroom. I reassured her that we were nearly there and I would give her prescribed oxygen as soon as possible. When we got back to her bed I tried to put the oxygen mask on her but she became very agitated and began pulling the mask off. Her colour changed and it was then I realized something was critically wrong. I stayed with her and called for assistance. The medical team arrived within minutes. During her subsequent resuscitation and examination it transpired that Anne had suffered a pulmonary embolism (PE).
2 How does it make you feel (as a nurse)?	I felt very bad initially that I may have missed something and perhaps I should have called for help sooner instead of assuming Anne was just short of breath in her usual way.
3 Evaluate: what was good or bad about the experience?	After the incident the ward nurses asked me what had happened and I explained. I felt guilty that moving Anne was the wrong thing to do, and that I should have recognized the signs and symptoms of hypoxia

(continued overleaf)

Table 6.2 Continued

	sooner. But the staff nurses were very supportive and explained that the PE could have occurred at any time. I also felt supported by the medical team who thanked me for staying and supporting Anne. The nurses told me that I reacted well to the emergency situation and they also said that they felt I did everything possible within this situation. When Anne awoke she said she remembered what had happened and thanked me for my support. She had felt very scared at the time and said she was glad I was there holding her hand.
4 *Analyse: what sense can you make of what happened?*	At the time of the incident I could have delayed my response and tried to maintain and manage the situation myself for longer. But I strongly felt that something more serious was happening and I needed help. I could have left the patient and gone for help but in the interest of the patient's well-being I thought she wouldn't want to be left alone. When the team arrived I could have stepped back from the patient as other more experienced nurses were present, but because Anne was my patient I felt I had a part to play in her effective resuscitation.

| 5 Conclude | Overall, I felt I did well for my first experience of a resuscitation and now feel, having critically reflected on this incident, that areas have been highlighted that I could improve on should a similar situation occur in my future nursing career. |
| 6 Action: what would you do differently in the future? | If a similar situation arose again I would know to act quickly in relation to alerting the resuscitation team. I would also be more prepared for the team's arrival - such as pre-empting the need to monitor the patient's O_2 sats and BP. Knowing the patient's details was very important and this was one area that I was competent in. |

As a result, Stephanie chose two of the An Bord Altranais (2004) competencies: 'holistic approaches to care and the integration of knowledge' and 'interpersonal relationships' to describe her learning in relation to the experience and guide her subsequent reading (a sample of her portfolio entry is given below).

Such emergency situations are not uncommon in nursing practice and can be very daunting, particularly for novice nurses. While Stephanie's story had a positive outcome in terms of the patient's recovery and Stephanie's own learning, had she not reflected on the event the situation may have been deemed as just another stressful day on the medical ward. Her reflections enabled her to examine her competence in relation to the following field competencies (NMC 2010: 18).

- All nurses must use up-to-date knowledge and evidence to assess, plan, deliver and evaluate care, communicate findings, influence change and promote health and best practice. They must make person-centred, evidence-based judgements and decisions, in partnership with others involved in the care process, to ensure high quality care. They must be able to recognize when the complexity of clinical decisions requires specialist knowledge and expertise, and consult or refer accordingly.

- Adult nurses must recognize and respond to the changing needs of adults, families and carers during terminal illness.
- Adult nurses must recognize the early signs of illness in people of all ages. They must make accurate assessments and start appropriate and timely management of those who are acutely ill, at risk of clinical deterioration or who require emergency care.

What could have been missed without an in-depth reflection was Stephanie's ability and competence in terms of facing and managing her responsibility as a potential Registered Nurse (RN). According to Newton and McKenna (2007) graduate nurses are often unprepared at the completion of their nurse education programme to deal with and manage the responsibilities and challenges of the job. The reflective portfolio is therefore a very good tool for documenting and critiquing your journey and recognizing your ability as a competent reflective practitioner.

Stephanie's portfolio entry went like this.

In providing care for Anne I believe I provided holistic nursing care incorporating physical, social and psychological caring. Further reading of the related literature validated this for me.

Caring is considered a core concept of nursing despite the concept of caring remaining ambiguous. Having read Rodgers (2000), I found five identified attributes of caring within nursing that include relationships, actions, attitudes, acceptance and variability. In order to achieve effective care, nurses must succeed in each attribute with their patients' care. I noted that McEvoy and Duffy (2008) also suggest that for holistic care to *take place an authentic nurse-patient relationship must exist. I believe that my interpersonal relationship skills ensured that such a relationship had developed between myself and Anne. By providing holistic care I allowed Anne to express her wishes with regard to what she wanted to do. Anne was aware of her condition and prognosis, not to mention her capabilities, and she felt comfortable in mobilizing to the toilet, perhaps to maintain a sense of her own dignity.*

Having cared for Anne I was aware that she was a strong-willed person who wished to remain independent with her care and only asked for assistance when she really required it. During the incident I was fully aware of Anne's apprehension and I tried to focus on providing nursing care for her body and mind by keeping her calm, offering reassurance and physical support and relaying relevant information during the event.

I knew she felt suffocated by the O_2 mask, so I tried to calm her by gently holding it up to her face rather than forcing her to put it over her head. Had I left Anne alone or insisted she put the mask on I would have abandoned any concept of holistic care. But instead, I waited with her, encouraged and reassured her and calmly explained what was happening, what we thought was best for her to do and that her family were on the way to see her. Bearing in mind that Anne probably thought she was going to die at this moment, it was important to successfully provide holistic care. The fact that Anne informed me afterwards that she felt relieved to have had my support when she needed it is evidence that a culture that supports a therapeutic relationship can result in a sense of wholeness, harmony and healing (McEvoy and Duffy 2008).

Although physical care was of the utmost importance in this situation it was vital that Anne was also emotionally supported. Had the outcome been less successful she may have died in a state of fear and confusion or with a sense of abandonment.

Transitioning from student to staff nurse I now feel that I developed a sense of the whole person and intuitively was aware that physical care was not the only priority of nursing care required in this situation. Those that have successfully provided holistic nursing care have described the use of a non-rational and intuitive 'way of knowing' within their practice as contributing to a change in the art of nursing theory and practice (Agan 1987). I believe I achieved this competency in relation to this event and also that I have a lot more learning to do with regard to achieving and maintaining holistic approaches towards my nursing care.

Using reflection as part of an action plan to influence my future practice has helped me to learn and to analyse my personal nursing skills. Reflection has enabled me to look at 'what I did in the situation' and justify my actions to determine if I proficiently managed events and what influenced me to react in the way that I did.

I have since researched the area of caring for patients with a PE and educated myself about the condition and the complications. I am now aware of the signs and symptoms to monitor closely including hypotension, chest pain, haemorrhage, haematuria, faecal occult blood, headache and confusion (Reid 1999).

I will know in the future to be extremely cautious should any of these symptoms arise in other patients in my care. Furthermore,

I am confident that I monitored my patient closely - Anne displayed no adverse signs or symptoms that morning while I regularly repeated her clinical observations. With regard to the competencies 'interpersonal relationships' and 'holistic approaches to care and the integration of knowledge' I feel I successfully achieved both of these and have the confidence to continue such nursing care in other situations.

However, I do realize that achieving competency in one incident does not imply that I will always be competent. The transition from student to staff nurse continues to provide me with a mixture of feelings and emotions: excitement, confidence, responsibility and sometimes fear. However, the learning will never stop even when I become registered; nursing practice is a continuous cycle of learning. The responsibility of remaining competent lies in my hands and I will utilize every avenue available to achieve that competence and become the best nurse that I possibly can be.

What is evident in Stephanie's account is how reflection can make intuitive knowledge clear and enable nurses to further build on their practice as a result. Her reflective portfolio entry highlights an effective learning experience. Not only did Stephanie take her own feelings into consideration, she also researched the relevant literature to improve her nursing care of managing patients diagnosed with a PE. This reading enabled her to draw on her clinical experiences and relate her practice back to theory, thus advancing her knowledge, promoting high quality patient-centred care and enhancing her decision-making ability. The article that she read by Reid informed her that her feelings of guilt regarding the care she provided for this patient were unfounded. Stephanie's entry encouraged her to develop self-awareness and take charge of her lifelong learning as a consequence.

Writing up

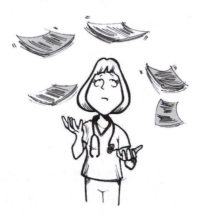

When you have identified an incident in your nursing practice which has had an impact on your care and which you feel would benefit from a process of structured reflection, you need to write it down 'in rough' while your memory of it is fresh (see below). Begin the reflection process by discussing your thoughts on the incident with your reflective friend, colleagues or facilitator. Then begin structured reflection in the same way Stephanie did. Use her example to help you if you need it, and start writing!

Tips for writing up your experience

● Write down your experience in your own words and then discuss it with your reflective friend, colleagues or facilitator. This discussion will help you begin your reflection.

● Use a model of reflection to analyse the experience and structure your writing.

- In order to relate your experience back to the theory, make reference to the literature or relevant policy documents in your write-up (as Stephanie did, above). Literature references are important, and useful for future reflection, so do try to read around your experience and include any useful references in your writing. You should also make a list of all the references you use in your portfolio giving the full details of each. If you are unsure how to do this, take a look at the reference list at the end of this chapter which shows the type of information that should be included. Your hospital librarian should be able to help you in your search once you have identified the key themes that emerge from your reflection.

As noted above, we suggest you begin to write your reflection on a critical incident using 'free writing': don't curtail yourself with any rules, just begin with a blank page and write down your thoughts on the incident as they come to you. The order does not matter at this stage. You can add more structure later, as Stephanie did.

Addressing the challenges

Reflective writing

Reflective writing requires the ability to think critically, and critical thinking can be difficult to articulate, teach and master. Critical thinking is not about being critically negative, but rather about providing an in-depth, holistic analysis, with the ultimate aim of developing your nursing practice. Critical reflection on practice can cause significant problems for nurses when trying to write up their reflective portfolio, usually because they find it hard to get started. Using a structured model of reflection (see Chapter 2) will always help, as will a selection of 'cues' to get your mind working (see Figure 6.2). The model

Aesthetic reflection

- What was I trying to achieve?

- Why did I respond as I did?

- What were the consequences of that for:

    the patient

    others

    myself?

- How was this person feeling?

- How did I know this?

Personal influencing factors

- How did I feel in this situation?

- What internal factors were influencing me?

Ethical consequences

- How did my actions match with my beliefs?

- What factors made me act in incongruent ways?

Empirical knowledge

- What knowledge did or should have informed me?

Reflexive learning

- How does this connect with previous experiences?

- Could I handle this better in similar situations?

- What would be the consequences of alternative actions for:

    the patient

    others

    myself?

- How do I feel about this experience?

- Can I support myself and others better as a consequence?

- Has this changed my way of knowing?

Figure 6.2 Cue questions for reflection (Johns 1995).

developed by Johns (1995), based on Carper's 'fundamental patterns of knowing' (1978) focuses on revealing the salient issues that often arise in nursing practice and clarifying the knowledge that guides that practice. The model uses five cues relating to aesthetic knowledge (i.e. the 'art' of nursing), personal knowledge, ethical knowledge, empirical knowledge and reflexive knowledge, which are then subdivided into focused questions to promote detailed reflection. Engaging with your reflective friend should help you critique and refine your entry.

Reflective writing tips

● Be honest when writing down your experiences. Write it *as it is*, not *as you would like it to be*.

● Be spontaneous. Don't spend lots of time working out what you're going to write, just *write something down* and then reflect on what you have written.

● Use your own words and write in the first person ('I') throughout.

● Persevere in the face of difficulties; use evidence-based literature or resources offered by your colleagues and reflective friend.

As discussed in detail in Chapter 2 a reflective friend usually represents a helpful ally in the process of reflection. They may be a colleague, lay-friend or even an experienced facilitator who is internal or external to your area of practice, but with whom you have developed a trusting relationship. On the other hand, you may not be comfortable with having a colleague critique your practice in which case the cue questions provided above will be very useful when you engage in 'solo reflection'. However, as we have emphasized again and again in this book, there is generally no substitute for a good model of reflection to help you structure your reflective writing and give you a 'kick start'.

Difficulties with self-reflection

Ghaye (2007: 152) describes one student's experience of writing her reflective portfolio:

> As students we are expected to fill our portfolios with reflections on our nursing experiences, this includes writing about things that upset us, reflecting upon possible triggers and how we felt afterwards. I remember leaning against the door of the sluice with my fingers in my ears to drown out the sound of an elderly patient calling again and again for her dead mother, who she swore had just gone to the corner shop. I remember becoming nauseated when entering the room of a dying patient and being transported back to the age of 11 when I had experienced the same smell in my father's room at the hospice ... My husband and best friend are the only two people I wish to confide in. My feelings are private – yet I am expected to frame them in prose and submit them to my university.

As this extract demonstrates, portfolio development is often a daunting exercise and many people shy away from reflecting on their practice, often because they feel uncomfortable when asked to share personal reflections with a friend, or are faced with reflecting on an incident they found difficult. Your reflective friend can be made aware of your concerns and if you are ever asked to act as a critical companion it is always a good idea to share your own reflections with your colleague. Particularly when discussing sensitive

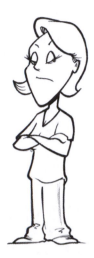

topics, nurses may find themselves becoming defensive about their practice and thus become cynical when trying to express personal opinions. On the other hand, remember that you *own* the portfolio and you *own* the reflection, so you choose how you want to write it.

Not everyone is a reflective thinker by nature, and for some nurses developing this skill can be difficult. In particular, if you have to focus on your fears and weaknesses as well as your strengths, you may perceive this activity initially as threatening. Ongoing reflective dialogue with a trusted colleague or using cue questions will help here, and like most skills, the more you practise the better you become. So don't be too disappointed if you struggle at first; persevere, and in time you will have a cohesive reflective portfolio that portrays you as a competent, caring nurse; a portfolio that you will be proud to show to others.

Ethical and legal issues

These were discussed in detail in Chapter 5, and they may in themselves present a barrier to your progress in building your portfolio. Briefly though, you need to be aware of current legislation and of course be familiar with your national and/or local code of practice and adhere to these in your portfolio. *Where* you work is also relevant: for example, if you work in the UK and were involved in an incident in relation to your care of a patient who underwent an abortion, this would be a perfectly valid portfolio entry for reflection and skill development. However, if you were involved in the same incident in another country it may not be.

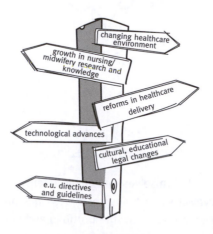

Your portfolio should demonstrate your professional decision-making ability, your accountability and your personal values as a nurse. At times you may experience conflict between you as a person and your professional values and ethics and it is worth critically examining your values to develop an understanding of how they affect your nursing care. Issues such as racism, ageism, sexual orientation, unprofessional and unethical practices or personal conflicts may all have an impact on your nursing practice. Don't let confrontation of such personal issues put you off writing for your portfolio: the exercise will ultimately be to your benefit as a professional practitioner.

If your portfolio is for personal and professional development only, there is *generally* no need to censor your reflections, but do remember that all documentation may be 'discoverable' through an order of the courts. It is more important to consider the legal and ethical issues inherent in your reflective accounts if you are presenting your portfolio for academic or accreditation purposes. Be aware that the assessor is more than likely to be a professional nurse and as such, has a legal obligation and professional responsibility to report any illegal or unethical practice you may have written about.

In order to prevent legal and ethical considerations from becoming a barrier to writing up your portfolio, it helps to bear in mind the following (Jasper 2003: 192):

- the type of language you use when referring to others;
- the way in which you report your actions from practice;
- the way in which you report that you have treated others;
- the consideration you give to respecting others and maintaining their dignity at all times;
- the general impression you give to others about your professional life and clinical practice.

It will also help, when considering an ethical or legal issue, to

- clarify the dilemma (e.g. by free writing, see above);
- gather additional data;
- identify your options;
- make a decision;
- act on your decision;
- evaluate the decision and its outcome as part of your critical reflection.

Finally, you need never have a dilemma about the following types of incident because they should *not* be included in a portfolio.

- Incidents that you are unsure about in relation to unethical or illegal practice.
- Incidents where a patient, relatives or others asked you to do something unethical or illegal.
- Incidents where you observed a peer or supervisor do something you perceived as unethical or illegal.
- Boundary issues (supervisor/supervisee; patient/nurse).
- Incidents where you failed to perform your duties of care.

All such incidents should of course be reported using the correct official channels and in line with local/national codes of practice.

Conclusion

In this chapter we discussed the concept of competence and nursing competencies and presented you with some examples from a nurse's ongoing portfolio showing how she progressed from her initial thoughts on an incident to structuring those thoughts using a model of reflection.

We also discussed some of the challenges nurses face when they begin to write up their portfolio – choosing a relevant incident, developing a reflective writing style and dealing with ethical and legal issues that may be inherent in the incident.

Summary

- Sections and subsections structured around core competencies form the backbone of your portfolio.
- Incidents for reflection can be the ordinary and regular experiences in practice, not just those that are traumatic or memorable.
- Use free writing to outline your chosen incident.
- Discuss your thoughts with your reflective friend if appropriate.
- Structure your writing using a model of reflection.
- The more you practise reflective writing the better you will become.
- Challenges and obstacles *can* be overcome.

References

Agan, R.D. (1987) Intuitive knowing as a dimension of nursing, *Advanced Nursing Science,* 10(1): 63–70.

An Bord Altranais (2000) *The Scope of Nursing and Midwifery Practice Framework*. Dublin: An Bord Altranais.

An Bord Altranais (2004) *Requirements and Standards for Nurse Registration Education Programmes*. Dublin: An Bord Altranais.

Carper, B. (1978) Fundamental patterns of knowing in nursing, *Advances in Nursing Sciences*, 1(1): 13–23.

Ghaye, T. (2007) Is reflective practice ethical? (The case of the reflective portfolio), *Reflective Practice*, 8(2): 151–62.

Gibbs, G. (1988) *Learning by Doing: A Guide to Teaching Learning Methods.* Oxford: Oxford Brookes University.

Girot E.A. (1993) Assessment of competence in clinical practice: a phenomenological approach, *Journal of Advanced Nursing*, 18(1): 114–19.

Jasper, M. (2003) *Beginning Reflective Practice*. Cheltenham: Nelson Thornes.

Johns, C. (1995) Framing learning through reflection within Carper's fundamental ways of knowing in nursing, *Journal of Advanced Nursing*, 22(2): 226–34.

McEvoy, L. and Duffy, A. (2008) Holistic practice – a concept analysis, *Nurse Education in Practice*, 8: 412–19.

NCNM (National Council for the Professional Development of Nursing and Midwifery) (2008a) *Framework for the Establishment of Clinical Nurse/Midwife Specialist Posts*, 4th edn. Dublin: NCNM.

NCNM (National Council for the Professional Development of Nursing and Midwifery) (2008b) *Framework for the Establishment of Advanced Nurse Practitioner and Advanced Midwife Practitioner Posts*, 4th edn. Dublin: NCNM.

Newton, J.M. and McKenna, L. (2007) The transitional journey through the graduate year: a focus group study, *International Journal of Nursing Studies*, 44(7): 1231–7.

NMC (Nursing and Midwifery Council) (2010) *Standards for Pre-registration Nursing Education*. London: NMC.

Reid, E. (1999) Pulmonary embolism: an overview of treatment and nursing issues, *British Journal of Nursing*, 8(20): 1373–8.

Rodgers, B.L. (2000) *Concept Development in Nursing: Foundations, Techniques, and Applications*, 2nd edn. Philadelphia, PA: W.B. Saunders.

Rush, D., McCarthy, G. and Cronin, C. (2000) *Report on Nursing Management*. Dublin: Office for Health Management.

Storey, L. (2001) *The Concept of Competence*. Proceedings of the Assessment of Competence Conference, Dublin, 13–14 September.

UKCC (United Kingdom Central Council for Nursing Midwifery and Health Visiting) (1999) *Fitness for Practice: The UKCC Commission for Nursing and Midwifery Education*. London: UKCC.

Valloze, J. (2009) Competence: a concept analysis, *Teaching and Learning in Nursing*, 4: 115–18.

WHO (World Health Organization) (1988) *Learning to Work Together for Health. Report of a WHO Study Group on Multi-professional Education for Health Personnel*. Geneva: WHO.

Zhang, Z., Luk, W., Arthur, D. and Wong, T. (2001) Nursing competencies: personal characteristics contributing to effective nursing performance, *Journal of Advanced Nursing*, 33(4): 467–74.

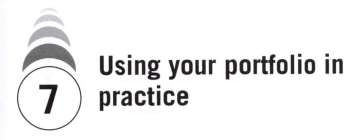

Using your portfolio in practice

7

By the end of this chapter you will:

- ○ Understand where your portfolio fits into your practice.
- ○ Appreciate how a portfolio is a 'living record'.
- ○ Be aware of how to widen your experience.
- ○ Understand how portfolios can help with accreditation.
- ○ Understand how you can use your portfolio to support change.
- ○ Understand how useful a 'field diary' can be.
- ○ Be aware of personal development plans.

This chapter explores using your nursing portfolio in practice. It also examines how your clinical practice can contribute directly to your portfolio, rather than the portfolio being seen simply as an academic exercise.

Where does it fit?

Historically, national regulatory bodies have prescribed and outlined the core content required of nurse preparation syllabi, and have defined the parameters of practice to ensure that practitioners are educated to and operate at the highest possible standards. More recent approaches to ongoing nurse registration in the UK, USA and Australia require greater emphasis on continuous professional development (CPD). The basis for this concern with standards and nurse education is patient safety and effective patient outcomes. Continuing competency, CPD and portfolio development are seen as integral to this.

In addition, nurses are becoming increasingly interested in mechanisms for ongoing professional development so as to keep up to date with modern thinking and develop their nursing competence on an ongoing basis. Competence is no longer thought of as a fixed entity whereby a nurse was deemed competent 'unless proven otherwise' but rather as something fluid and, crucially, *evolving*. Clinical competence evolves not only because of your personal characteristics, skills and knowledge, but as a result of the challenges you face in the workplace such as complex healthcare needs and mastering new technologies.

As a nurse, in addition to professional requirements for CPD, you will undoubtedly have recognized that continually maintaining and developing your competence in practice is a challenge. This is where the portfolio fits in. By reflecting on your own learning and identifying and planning for new learning experiences you can develop and maintain your competence, suited to your personal learning needs.

Remember!

The portfolio is a vehicle that assists you in addressing your ongoing learning needs.

The portfolio as a living record

Your portfolio is a living record of your clinical professional development, whatever your speciality, be it general or adult nursing, psychiatry, midwifery, intellectual disability nursing or children's nursing. It paints a picture of how you practise as a professional nurse, allowing you to identify effective practice, build on your strengths and work on your weaknesses. Portfolios are initially created for numerous reasons including for accreditation or promotional purposes, for academic assessment and for assisting ongoing professional development. Many nurses compile a portfolio for more than one of these reasons. Whatever the reason, as time goes by, if you have created and maintained a good portfolio, you will begin to notice that your *intuitive ability* improves. You will be able to anticipate situations and be better able to deal with them as a result. Such intuitive ability relates to Carper's (1978) 'patterns of knowing in nursing' which embrace four of the distinct areas that were first introduced in Chapter 6: empirics (the science and knowledge base of nursing); aesthetics (the 'art' of nursing); 'personal knowing' and 'ethical knowing'. As your practice proceeds, your portfolio will enhance your development in these areas and you in turn can use *them* to enhance your portfolio in a manner that goes beyond the purely competence-based approach we have advocated so far. Such a development of your portfolio, based on experience in practice, reinforces the fact that the portfolio is a *living record* of your journey as a professional nurse.

Widening your experience

Maintaining your portfolio will encourage you to engage in wider reading (see Chapter 6) and to attend other learning opportunities such as formal courses and conferences. Naturally, the portfolio will in turn be enriched by what you bring back from such activities.

If you are unfamiliar with the concept of *critical reading*, which is necessary for you to properly analyse and apply the content of published work to your practice, you will find the 'learning zones' provided by the *Nursing Standard* extremely helpful in setting you on your way. These are available at http://nursingstandard.rcnpublishing.co.uk/ and access is by subscription. The benefit of the learning zone approach is that it gives you a simple and focused introduction to reading around a particular subject and also invites nurses to submit a *practice profile* to the journal. As a result you can read other nurses' submissions, which can be very helpful in learning about the experience of others and seeing the type of writing style they adopt. The practice profiles also provide PREP solutions to help you with your CPD. Certificates of achievement form part of the learning zone process, and these can form excellent artefacts for addition to your portfolio. Another learning zone that may be a helpful resource for your professional and portfolio development is the RCN zone. This is a free online service aimed at helping RCN members with their CPD and professional portfolio management, available at www.rcn.org.uk/members/learningzone.php

Always try to have a focus and a structure to your additional learning and reading. In addition to making your portfolio unwieldy, random 'certificate-gathering' or reading (i.e. not related to a particular personal learning need) is counterproductive and can lead to stress because you are trying to do too much. Do not attend courses and read journals just for the sake of it, but always have your personal learning needs at the forefront of your mind.

If you think back to the example of David Omotosa in Chapter 4 (see pp. 84–91), his reading as a result of his reflection was very focused in the area of dementia and nurse–patient relationships. He could also expand his reading into other related areas such as dignity and quality of life. This type of focused learning and reading in key areas is much more valuable that an *ad hoc* approach.

Wherever you go for your information, always try to make use of high quality peer-reviewed journal papers. A good way to access and research these is via a dedicated online database such as:

- CINAHL (Cumulative Index to Nursing and Allied Health Literature)
- MEDLINE/Pubmed
- Cochrane Database
- ERIC
- PSYLIT

Such databases will enable you to engage in a literature search, which is always the best starting point when researching a particular aspect of practice. Although it is beyond the scope of this book to examine the full process of literature search and review, some basic principles that you may find helpful are:

- Choose your topic
- Brainstorm the topic to identify key questions within the area
- Narrow down your chosen topic to one or two questions/problems in the area
- From this narrowing-down process select key words to use in your search
- Use these key words as the basis for your search
- Retrieve available articles for reading

The same basic principles apply if you are engaging in a search of paper-based archives such as your local hospital library.

Accreditation

Your portfolio can be used for accreditation of prior experiential learning (APEL), an academic award you can obtain for previously-acquired learning from your clinical experience which has not been previously assessed or certificated. You can also gain accreditation through work-based learning (WBL) which relates to planned learning negotiated between an individual, employer and an academic institution that can be considered for an academic award in the future.

Thus your portfolio plays an important part in your beginning to bridge the 'theory–practice gap' that so many academics talk about. Your nursing practice will become more evidenced-based and the knowledge you gain from reading the literature will help address issues that you may previously have considered 'swampy' (Schön 1983). In turn, as your practice becomes more evidenced-based, your nursing skills will be enriched as a result.

Experiencing and implementing change

Your portfolio will eventually become like a photo album. Have you ever looked at an old photo collection and thought to yourself, 'Look how much I've changed?' The same should apply when you revisit your portfolio entries. You will be able to see a metamorphosis of yourself over time. Skills such as reflection, critical thinking and creative writing will have emerged and developed and your confidence and competence improved. It truly is a transformative process and most nurses who have produced and maintained a portfolio say that despite the hard work they have experienced a wonderful journey of self-development. Not only that, but your portfolio has the power to *implement change*. It can act as a catalyst for changing either yourself or an area of your nursing practice that requires attention (David gives a good example of this in Chapter 4). A portfolio can also be extended to create a 'team' or 'departmental'

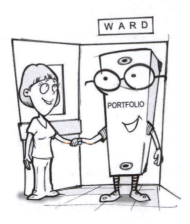

portfolio. Rassin *et al.* (2006) recommend such a portfolio for assessing, imple-menting and evaluating departmental practices. In such a portfolio, staff CVs are kept together in one section, and the philosophy of the unit, job descrip-tions and so on are allocated to other sections. Further sections could focus on staff development activities and achievements, student nurses and patient care, perhaps even including a selection containing patient information leaf-lets, especially if staff members have designed or created them.

For such a portfolio to be successful (and as importantly, *useful*) you need to be collaborative and decide together on the aims and objectives of the departmental portfolio. Speak with your colleagues and your manager about taking your departmental portfolio into practice. Since Together Everyone Achieves More, encouraging a TEAM approach is essential. A depart-mental portfolio is a creative way of encouraging staff to embrace and engage in the process of change, and in practice development and improvement.

Even if your nursing colleagues are not yet interested in developing a departmental portfolio, you can (and should) attempt to look at how you can use your own portfolio to improve patient care. Once you have mastered the skill of reflecting on your own practice, you can start to 'step outside' that practice and look at what you can achieve by, for example, teaching others the skills of reflection and encouraging them to develop their own portfolios. Nervousness about the whole concept of portfolios may be the reason why your colleagues are shying away from the idea of a departmental portfolio. If so, your encouragement may help them to regard the idea with less alarm and more enthusiasm.

Another way of bringing your portfolio into practice is by helping students develop their reflective skills and clinical portfolios. Because the students, one hopes, will be up-to-date with the literature, particularly in relation to reflective practice, portfolio development and the nursing-related competencies, you will most likely have as much to learn from them as they have from you. This is where learning becomes a two-way process – you have as much to give as to receive and, between you, you can exchange your 'know how knowledge' (borne from practical experience) with their 'know that knowledge' (borne from up-to-date study) to become both 'know that' and 'know how' nurses!

Helping others and asking for help

Most nurses come to the profession because they want to help others. The portfolio development process also allows you to help yourself, and as a consequence to be more effective in the way you help others. On those occasions when you feel oppressed in your practice, perhaps as a result of some of the barriers we have discussed in this book, your by now trusted reflective friend, your developing critical thinking skills and your emerging evidence-based portfolio offer an ideal way to help yourself out of such a situation, at the same time improving as a nurse and as a result increasing the quality of patient care you are able to offer.

As an enhancement of the reflective processes we have discussed throughout this book, you may wish to consider what is known as 'guided reflection'. Think of this as a kind of step up from the more informal sessions you engage in with your reflective friend (who may, indeed, be a lay-person in any case). Your partner in this type of exercise is usually referred to as a 'facilitator' and will usually have some considerable experience in guiding the reflective process. Facilitated reflection sessions should normally not be any longer than an hour, because the process can be mentally and even emotionally taxing.

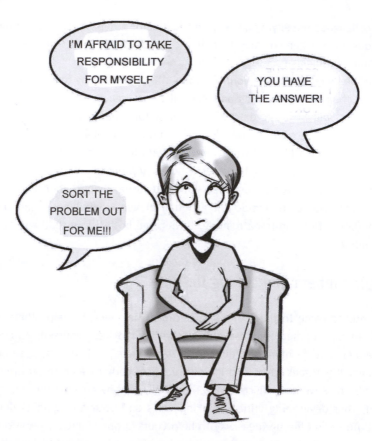

You must be prepared for what may unfold during such sessions, and you will find reading Duffy (2008) helpful. Not every guided reflection session will go well, and under such circumstances your facilitator may decide to adjourn the session. This is perfectly acceptable and indeed it is better to stop than to keep going and damage your relationship. It may simply be that you and your colleague have different views on the issue being discussed and need 'time out' to think more about each other's perspective before returning to the process. In some cases you may both decide that the guided reflection sessions are not fruitful (perhaps you simply chose the wrong person to guide you), and this is also fine.

Keeping a diary

Unfortunately nursing practice is often so busy you may find that after a 12-hour shift you are far too tired to sit down and reflect on any given incident. Not only that, but your family and social life will always, understandably, come first over reflective exercises, portfolios and the like. We understand that developing a portfolio is time-consuming. In an ideal world protected 'reflective time' would be made available to every nurse as part of their working hours and, on that basis, the development of a professional portfolio could be made a compulsory aspect of professional practice. However, as things stand at the moment, such a development is unlikely, so as we have discussed in previous chapters, the development of your portfolio is entirely down to you and must take place in your own time.

In addition to our suggestion of allocating your own 'protected time' in which you can devote yourself to the valuable work of portfolio development and personal reflection, you may find it helpful to keep a 'diary' in the form of field notes, to which you can refer at a later date and which contains your immediate thoughts on any aspect of your practice you deem to be worthy of note. A good example is the recording, in rough, of a critical incident at work, as soon as you finish your shift. (Remember that 'critical incident' means an event that is critical to *you*, not necessarily a major clinical crisis such as a patient suffering a PE, for example. In many cases something far more mundane may have 'critical' status in terms of its impact on you and your developing professional practice.) If you choose to keep a diary or field-note record, remember that issues relating to confidentiality, legality and ethics (see Chapter 5) remain the same.

Remember!

Do not use names or details in your diary that could identify anyone involved in the situation you are recording.

A further advantage of keeping a diary is that you can take it to work and if you have time (e.g. on a night shift) make brief notes of your feelings, actions and concerns at the time and expand upon them later. We recommend a hardback notebook, small enough to keep with you or in your locker at work.

Many of your entries are likely to be a combination of notes made during a shift and further thoughts jotted down when at home. The example below shows you what we mean, with the first three entries made during a quiet point on a shift and the last three made after work. You can see immediately that there is rich material here for further reflection and development into a useful portfolio entry for the nurse concerned.

Date: 16 July, late shift

What happened?

Pt fell out of bed while trying to climb over the cot sides and was lying on the floor for 10 mins. He was in a single room and was unable to call for help because his door was closed. We were short staffed and both my two colleagues and I were changing an incontinent patient at the time of the incident. A visitor passed the room and heard him calling and then alerted us.

My feelings

I'm so embarrassed and angry and ashamed and upset for the patient.

My actions

Assessed patient, called Dr and Nursing Admin, filled out incident form, patient had to have an x-ray and sustained a

---

fractured left hip. It took the rest of the evening to attend to the patient's needs. We then moved him to the main ward. He was furious, because he is a private patient and wanted his own room and privacy.

Date: 17 July

Return to my feelings

Even more annoyed now at the patient - he should have waited until we were able to assist him, rather than try to get out of bed himself.

Why am I concerned?

Annoyed at me also, as nurse in charge of shift, for not making a better assessment of Mr J. If a thorough nursing assessment was made of Mr J. in the first instance we may have realized he was not suitable for a private room. Cot sides should also not have been in place - this is not evidence-based practice. Patient's safety was not prioritized.

Action plan

Need to read article regarding use of cot sides. Go to library in morning. Need to speak to staff re: accurately assessing patients prior to allocating them to a single room.

Theme: accountability - legal and ethical practitioner

You should find that making notes like those shown in the example is cathartic and will also help to make what happened clearer in your mind. Brief after-shift reflections help to make you more objective about your feelings and also, as in this case, to vent any pent up anger or frustration that might otherwise cloud a session of full reflection on an incident at a later date.

The personal development plan

Your nursing portfolio benefits you more than anyone else. By bringing your learning to life, you should feel more motivated to reflect, analyse, research and practise nursing using an evidence-based approach. This 'personal audit' of your practice will over time result in improvements in your standards of patient care, entice you to engage in continued learning and enhance your personal and professional development. You will find yourself identifying gaps in your knowledge and bridging those gaps by reading and engaging in other learning activities. The new learning is then applied to your clinical practice, and a fresh round of reflection and development begins.

When you have completed the first cycle of your portfolio, apart from having cause for celebration, you will be in a position to create a personal development plan (PDP) to help you to structure your long-term learning and career plans (see Table 7.1).

Your PDP will help to form the basis of a logical summary for your portfolio. It makes sense that when you have completed your first cycle of portfolio development, you should examine this experience as a whole, summarize it and identify where you need to go next in terms of your learning and career goals. You will recall that in Chapter 2 we suggested you give thought to the following questions in the context of starting your portfolio:

- Where have I been?
- Where am I now?
- Where would I like to be?
- How will I get there?

At the completion of your portfolio you should give consideration to these questions again as you plan your future action. In conjunction with the framework shown in Table 7.1, this will guide you towards outlining your PDP.

Table 7.1 Example of a personal development plan (PDP)

Step	Evidence
Step 1 Previous experience	Write a summary of your nursing experiences, perhaps referring to the section within your portfolio where your clinical experience is listed and/or the section containing your CV.
Step 2 Learning from experience	Summarize your overall learning following reflecting within the portfolio, discussions with a reflective friend and reviewing the literature/policy documents.
Step 3 Demonstrate competence	Summarize your evidence for your chosen elements of clinical competencies or practice that you identified within your subsections.
Step 4 Learning needs	Document your learning needs on completion of the portfolio. This forms the basis of the PDP.
Step 5 Developing a learning programme	Write an account of what you need to do to achieve your PDP, and what you now need to do in order to continuously progress. This could be continued learning through your portfolio, more attendance at study events, more reading on key topics or something more structured such as enrolling for a degree, master's or higher degree programme of study.

Conclusion

Throughout this book we have explained in detail the practical manner in which you can develop your personal and professional portfolio to showcase your achievements and nursing life experience. You don't need to be a student or to be undertaking a nurse education programme to begin this journey; in fact all you need is a folder, paper, pen, small hardback notebook, perhaps a reflective friend and the heart and commitment to begin and engage in the process.

In this book we have shown you how to use the 'tools of the trade': the skills of reflection, reflective and critical writing, choosing and working with a reflective friend, and building your portfolio from the 'bottom up' using sections, subsections and a suitable framework based, for example, on core nursing competencies. We have also discussed alternative formats for your portfolio, including the e-portfolio, and examined potential barriers to your progress, suggesting ways in which these can be overcome and, we hope, demonstrating the enormous benefits that building a reflective portfolio can bring.

Although there continues to be a small number of antagonists sitting on the sidelines, criticizing both reflection and portfolio development, the best reason they can offer for their argument seems to be insufficient empirical evidence to demonstrate the effectiveness of reflection on practice and warrant its continued use in nursing. However, we believe these arguments are weak, and now outdated. Reflection as a concept has been around for over 100 years (Dewey 1933) and will remain with us for a long time to come. In the words of Johns and Freshwater (1998: x), reflective practice as a therapeutic process gives us 'wings to soar as we emerge from our cocoons to make a holistic journey of personal transformation and growth'.

We hope you have been encouraged to begin that journey soon.

Summary

- Your portfolio is an integral component of your CPD.
- Keeping a portfolio will enhance your intuitive practice over time.
- Keeping a portfolio will stimulate you to engage in wider reading and other learning opportunities.
- Portfolios can contribute to accreditation (e.g. APEL, WBL).
- Sharing your learning with others is a useful way of learning yourself.
- Keep a diary to build up potential material for your portfolio.
- When you complete the first 'cycle' of your portfolio, consider mapping out a PDP for the future.

References

Carper, B. (1978) Fundamental patterns of knowing in nursing, *Advances in Nursing Sciences*, 1(1): 13–23.

Dewey, J. (1933) *How We Think*. Boston, MA: J.C. Heath.

Duffy, A. (2008) Guided reflection: a discussion of the essential components, *British Journal of Nursing*, 17(5): 334–9.

Johns, C. and Freshwater, D. (eds) (1998) *Transforming Nursing Through Reflective Practice*. London: Blackwell Science.

Rassin, M., Silner, D. and Ehrenfeld, M. (2006) Departmental portfolio in nursing: an advanced instrument, *Nurse Education in Practice*, 6(1): 55–60.

Schön, D. (1983) *The Reflective Practitioner*. London: Temple Smith.

References

Index

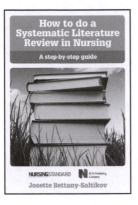

**HOW TO DO A SYSTEMATIC
LITERATURE REVIEW IN NURSING
A step-by-step guide**

Josette Bettany-Saltikov

9780335242276 (Paperback)
January 2012

eBook also available

This is a step-by-step guide to doing a literature review in
nursing that takes you through every step of the process from
start to finish. From writing your review question to writing up
your review, this practical book is the perfect workbook
companion if you are doing your first literature review for study
or clinical practice improvement.

The book features extracts from real literature reviews to help
illustrate good practice as well as the pitfalls to avoid. Full of
practical explanations this book will be invaluable at every
stage. A must buy!

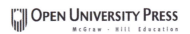
OPEN UNIVERSITY PRESS
McGraw - Hill Education

www.openup.co.uk